The
INSECURE GIRL'S
Handbook

The
INSECURE GIRL'S
Handbook

Join the Club,
then learn how to leave it!

OLIVIA PURVIS

SEVEN DIALS

First published in Great Britain in 2020 by Seven Dials,
This paperback edition published in 2023 by Seven Dials
an imprint of The Orion Publishing Group Ltd
Carmelite House, 50 Victoria Embankment
London EC4Y 0DZ

An Hachette UK Company

1 3 5 7 9 10 8 6 4 2

ISBN (Paperback) 978 1 8418 8388 5
ISBN (eBook) 978 1 8418 8389 2

Printed and bound in Great Britain by Clays Ltd, Elcograf, S.p.A

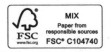

www.orionbooks.co.uk

For Mum and Dad – the original nervous Purvises.

I love you.

Contents

Introduction

You're on a boat with Emma Watson, Beyoncé, Michelle Obama and Meryl Streep. Imagine! Is this a P&O celebrity cruise special? No! This is HMS *Insecurity* – and we're all riding it together. Some of us hop off at different ports, but if 'we're all in the same boat' ever applies, ladies, I'm pretty sure it's right about now. Because yes, they've felt like this too.

. . . .

'I, as a twenty-one-year-old, was riddled with insecurity and self-critiquing. Some of my friends still are. I realised that I didn't like friends taking photos of me when I wasn't working and I actually got in a fight about this issue. And I wondered, why is this bothering me? Why does this make me so insecure? And I realised it's because I can't even reconcile myself with my own image on the front of these magazines.'[1]

EMMA WATSON, feminist, activist
and actor extraordinaire

'After the birth of my first child, I believed in the things society said about how my body should look. I put pressure on myself to lose all the baby weight in three months, and scheduled a small tour to assure I would do it. Looking back, that was crazy.'[2]

BEYONCÉ, so successful she doesn't use a surname

'At this point, I'd been First Lady for just over two months. In different moments, I'd felt overwhelmed by the pace, unworthy of the glamour, anxious about our children, and uncertain of my purpose.'[3]

MICHELLE OBAMA, no introduction needed

'Oh, I'm sure that my career has been wonderful, and people talk about accolades and such, but somehow that doesn't register with me. My mother used to say to me, "Why don't you enjoy it more? Some people would give an arm and a leg to walk down the red carpet at a movie premiere, why can't you enjoy it?" But I just don't get into it, I'm afraid. I have my own doubts, worries and insecurities, and that's what I fixate on.'[4]

MERYL STREEP, often described as the best actor of her generation

. . . .

If I were going to add in my own quote (for a minor Beyoncé moment) it would probably be something like:

. . . .

'Throughout my career, it's always seemed that if you have followers (one type of "success currency" with a terrible exchange rate) then you can't be insecure. As if a series of likes and well-curated photographs could be cashed in for unflappable confidence.'

LIV PURVIS, blog writer, podcast host and author,
who would probably introduce herself nervously
as 'a jack-of-all-trades' instead

. . . .

And, if I'm being honest, the thought of writing a book about insecurity made me feel insecure. In fact, whenever I approach a new project I'm always riddled with self-doubt: Am I good enough? What if people don't like it? Do people care about what I have to say? How did I manage this? But feeling insecure and uncertain is unfortunately common-place in the lives of modern women and men everywhere; a national report on the state of self-esteem (commissioned by the Dove Self-Esteem Fund) discovered that 62 per cent of girls feel insecure or not sure of themselves, and seven out of ten believe they aren't good enough or 'don't mea-sure up' in some way.[5] It's much bigger than just a word – it's something that is stirred by new experiences; old ex-periences; new relationships; unpredictable everyday chal-lenges; and sometimes by the simple belief that someone else could be doing it a lot better. Insecurity comes when you both least and most expect it – sometimes it feels like it never gets easier to manage, and it can be one of the most crippling and overwhelming feelings to overcome. Insecurity can make everyone – you, the woman next to you on the train, the girl who served you your coffee this morning, and the woman you had a meeting with this afternoon – doubt their capabilities.

At what age did you start feeling insecure?

Under 13: 43% I 13–17: 46% I 18–24: 9% I 25–34: 2% I Don't know: <1%

The reality is, no matter who you are – no matter how rich, beautiful, successful or happy – insecurity is a universal experience. Whether it's attacks of self-doubt, worries over what people think of you, or a general lack of confidence, the truth is we've all been part of The Insecure Girls' Club at one point or another. When I started The Insecure Girls' Club on Instagram in 2018, my insecurities were at their prime. As a twenty-five-year-old woman shrouded in self-doubt, I'd had endless conversations with friends about the insecurities and worries we shared, and we seemed to pass them off so casually that I wondered if feeling wobbly was just a natural course that we all had to take. But I knew it

---

* These percentages are taken from an online survey of 461 women we carried out specifically for this book. All percentages included in these boxes relate to this survey.

wasn't just me and my direct circle feeling like this. The conversation had the potential to be a lot bigger and more impactful than a few women around a table with some lemonade and wine – which is when I started the page @TheInsecureGirlsClub. Since then, I've learnt that no matter how uncertain or insecure you're feeling, you're never alone. Some of the most confident, able and success-ful women I know have spoken to me about the complex edifices of insecurity. It doesn't matter how high-achieving they appear (and are) from the outside; they've all ques-tioned at one point or another where they are in life and whether they're good enough.

. . . .

'I remember looking in the mirror and being completely disappointed by the way I looked. I never saw anyone in the media who looked like me. They all represented an ideal that was completely unobtainable.'

STEPHANIE, Chelmsford

. . . .

It never fails to surprise me when I'm reminded just how common this emotion is. And isn't that pretty much what it is – an emotion? Just like anger, sadness and joy, insecurity is something we all *feel*. If Queen Bey can feel insecure about her next performance (whilst winning endless awards), and a certain Ms Chung can feel out of her depth and wor-ried about people pleasing (which she has spoken about openly),[6] then surely we can acknowledge that self-doubt is something women everywhere are battling.

How many times have you left a dinner, or a party with new friends, or a work meeting that's pushed you out of your comfort zone, and switched into a self-critical mode of endless over-analysing? It happened to me last week after a beautiful press dinner with a handful of women I didn't know particularly well. Finding something that could be wrong and creating a narrative to construct a problem to probe ourselves with is all too easy: 'Did I come across as too loud and overbearing?', 'Did I not talk enough?', 'I wonder if that thing I said offended that girl?', 'Oh God, why did I laugh at my own jokes so much?'. Negative self-talk is just the tip of the iceberg when it comes to insecurity, and the time we spend second-guessing our own judgements and actions could really be spent doing something far more positive and productive. I left that work dinner last week and messaged one of my best friends saying: 'Oh God, was I really annoying?' She replied: 'No – but so what if you were?'

I was at my most insecure when I'd just dropped out of university. I'd been studying English and communication studies, and although I loved the city I was in, I had about as much excitement and passion for the course as I did watching Sunday afternoon snooker on TV (very little). It wasn't what I'd signed up for, and I felt overwhelmed about who I'd let down, who I'd disappointed and what I'd do next. If I wasn't going to have 'BA Hons' next to my name, how would I define myself when people asked me what I was doing? Would I be known as a drop-out until I was eighty? Was my lack of UCAS kudos going to follow me around forever?

I frantically applied for courses at the London College of Fashion (the pinnacle of status in the industry, to yours truly), and after not getting in with a terrible nerve-fuelled essay, I felt so unconfident in my abilities. All the successful women in fashion I'd heard of had gone to university – suddenly I felt lost and out of my depth. But fast-forward to today, and it's safe to say I made the right decision. Running two businesses, creating a team of wonderful women and co-hosting a podcast (*The Fringe of It*, with my pal Charlotte Jacklin) might never have happened had I not decided to go with my gut all those years ago. Yet this feeling is something that continues to rear its ugly head, time and time again – no matter how well *on paper* I appear to be doing. I've lost count of the number of times I've felt like I'm not working hard enough, just because I'm working differently from someone else. What I can say with total confidence, however, is that it's 100 per cent possible to learn how to challenge these feelings and handle them better, so they don't ruin your day.

I don't believe there's ever a point in life where we feel successful enough, that we've 'made it' – unless of course we make it for ourselves. It's about creating personal measures of success that are attainable and realising that success doesn't have an expiry date. Sharing and celebrating the small successes in life and realising it's OK to be your own spokesperson can be the key to serious self-validation. It's when we come together in a group and talk about these mutual concerns that we really start becoming easier on and kinder to ourselves, and realise that ultimately, we are all the same.

So, welcome to The Insecure Girls' Club – we are so very happy to have you as part of the family, and a community that's proved when one person is willing to talk about their insecurities, they open up an arena for thousands of women. This handbook will guide you through days when you don't feel able, confident or good enough to step up and get things done – through those universal experiences of insecurity that we all feel.

In these pages, you'll find tips, coping mechanisms and small pearls of wisdom, as well as peppy pick-me-up take-aways at the end of each chapter. I've included interviews with women who have a next-level understanding of different aspects of insecurity, and who share not only their first-hand experiences of some of the insecurities that touch us all, but also how they've faced these moments head-on, be it in their education, career or personal life. There are also plenty of wise, knowing words from other members of the club, showing that no matter how alone or silly you might feel voicing these concerns, you're never the only person feeling like this. You should never have to apologise, and these ladies have seen it from both sides – because there's always another side.

This book is a comforting hug, a reassuring smile and a pep talk, from one insecure girl to another, served in digestible chunks (when a two-for-one pizza offer just isn't going to cut it). It's a book you can come back to when you suddenly feel out of your depth or like you're a tiny fish swimming in a very large pond. It's a go-to support system filled with the voices of other insecure girls just like you, who also want to manage their anxiety better, stop imposter syndrome in its tracks, and halt the waves of self-doubt that unexpectedly flood their reality. Come back to these pages again and again when you need them. Make them dog-eared if you want to, and underline the things you'll want to come back to as freely as you wish. This book is yours. (Unless it's from your local library – then maybe hold off for the time being . . .)

So, here's to treating ourselves like we treat others, putting ourselves first, and being the secure and thoughtful women that we know we can be. If this nervous Purvis can create a toolkit to combat those insecurities and clip that self-doubt, then you can too. Hopefully these pages will make you realise that we are all worthy of taking up space, and that we often need to trust our own judgement and leave the worrying until later. It's for the girls just starting out in their careers (when 'no worries if not!' is our most used phrase), and the young women at the top of them too (when it's still our most used phrase). The girls worrying about making the leap to put something out there, and the ones who have been doing it for a while but feel like they've lost their mojo along the way. It will stop you from feeling that you're not doing things right on time on the unwritten road of life (which is as deep as I promise to get). As my sixteen-year-old self would have said after a *High School Musical* binge, 'We're All In This Together'! And even if it's me telling you that instead of Zac Efron and Vanessa Hudgens, I promise you we *can* do this together.

1

'You're so embarrassing':
one on one with your inner critic

Coping with the Simon Cowell voice inside
that's ready to cry out 'it's a no from me'

Although there are so many veins of insecurity that we
experience and endure to different degrees, at the heart of
all insecurity lies the big cheese: our inner critic. It appears
endlessly; whether within friendships, in our body image,
comparing ourselves to others, or just those day-to-day
worries – like trying to assert ourselves in the office, or
setting a boundary where we hadn't before. When we least
want or need it, the inner critic will be sure to appear, nar-
rating and advising; sparking self-doubt and flicking away
any scraps of confidence. It can feel overwhelming at times
and insignificant at others – but by being aware of that
critical voice, we can make a meaningful change to how
we treat ourselves going forward – not letting it dictate the
things we say to ourselves, especially when we're learning
how to harness tricky situations.

> **Was there a defining moment when you started feeling insecure?**
>
> 'Having a cleft lip, I became aware very early on that I had an obvious physical difference. I remember looking in the mirror and recognising that difference, and wishing it wasn't the case.'
>
> *Jess, Leicester*

I first experienced the feeling of insecurity when I was at primary school, around the age of eight, when someone kindly pointed out the shape and size of my ears – unintentionally planting a tiny insecurity seed with their words. I suddenly felt enormously aware of them – mentally agreeing with every 'big ears' or 'Dumbo' comment I was confronted with, even if it was from myself. When someone points out something about you that you feel conscious of, it becomes ten times easier for your inner critic to start buckling you with that insecurity too. Looking back now, it seems completely ridiculous. At the time, my real priorities were acquiring the full collection of Bratz dolls and wondering why my popcorn-scented gel pen didn't show up on white paper. (Who invents these things?!) To think that from such a young age I started to become aware of what I now recognise as 'flaws' seems ridiculous. (Especially in a world with white gel pens . . .)

I think my inner critic truly manifested when I was in sixth form. I was a Myspace-loving teenager with little to no online etiquette (nobody ever said in school that if someone declines your friend request more than five times, it's probably a no from them too), and there were times in my yellow jeans phase when insecurity would rear its head. But it was when I switched school for Years 12 and 13 that my insecurities became really apparent. I was surrounded by new faces, a new environment, and new teachers who didn't appreciate that I'd sooner lose every PC4PC (that's 'picture comment for picture comment', for anyone who grew up pre- or post-Myspace) or pound of phone credit than ever voluntarily answer a question in class. At one point I thought I had IBS because I was so nervous. Then there were the boys, of course – both revelatory and terrifying for someone who had previously been to an all-girls school and never wore make-up from Monday to Friday. And, as a seventeen-year-old, I didn't drink. As the only one at house parties, eighteenth birthdays and Reading Festival who didn't fancy touching a drop of alcohol, I felt acutely aware of being the 'odd one out' in a group of people – as if there was a spotlight on my social skills, when actually I'd have quite happily faded into a magnolia-painted background. This dripped into my (albeit brief) stint at university, and continues now in my twenty-something life as a self-employed woman.

Equally often, there isn't a significant 'Ah, so that was when I became hyper-critical of myself' moment; it's something that subtly appears in everyday life, built up from lots of smaller moments that we leave unquestioned and unmentioned.

We forget that nearly every other person around us experiences it in some capacity – wondering where this strange feeling came from, and who is responsible for it. So, when does insecurity begin? Sometimes it arises from embarrassing or challenging situations in the past, which leave a tiny imprint in your memory – from not-so-subtle comments about your dodgy outfit or food choices to friendship fall-outs and uncomfortable job interviews.

As well as these smaller moments, there are always going to be the unshakable ones that seemingly stay with you forever. Although just the thought of putting it on paper makes my hands clammy (sorry, Nan), I remember when an immature ex-boyfriend shouted 'HAIRY MUFF!' across the train platform at London Bridge – leaving a tomato-faced fifteen-year-old me thinking body hair was the antithesis of being a successful girlfriend, and that the only romantic endeavors I'd be destined for would be more suited to a (not so) sexy seventies film, where purple silk sheets and 'Help Yourself' by Tom Jones playing on repeat would reign supreme. How would I ever find love again? Who would ever look at me with desire and longing if I had a . . . *hairy muff*?

FUELLED BY EMOTION – 'WHY AM I LIKE THIS?!'

Whenever I wonder why these moments have such significance, I always think of my favourite Disney film, *Inside Out*. In case you haven't seen it (go watch it now!), it's set inside the head of a young girl called Riley, whose emotions are personified as characters – Joy, Sadness, Fear, Disgust and Anger – who decide what she says and does through a whizzy control board. The film is brilliant in so many ways, but when it comes to thinking about insecurity, it reminds me of our inner critic – how vocal it can be when we least need it and how our emotions are so intrinsically linked and heightened, feeding off each other. There's a scene where Fear becomes flustered and panicked, saying, 'Did you see that look? They're judging us!' when Riley is talking in front of her class; it's such a good example of how the inner critic seems like it's protecting us, but is actually inciting panic or worry instead. We're more likely to give ourselves praise when we're feeling joyful, and certainly more inclined to give ourselves a knock when we're feeling sadness, fear or anger.

How often do you worry about what others think?

Several times a day: 54% I Several times a week: 22% I Once a day: 14% I Once a week: 8% I Once a month: 1% I Never: <1%

Sometimes, all it takes is one tiny tumble for our brain to catastrophise everything within that moment and every similar experience in the future. Like the hyperbolic teenage echoes of 'This has ruined my life' that suddenly appear when you crack a joke to a silent group, or you overhear someone saying, 'Oh, she was just a bit much today' – or worse, 'Nope, I did hear you first time' after that terrible joke. I remember so many occasions as a teenager when something ridiculous happened and I was certain that it would follow me into my adult life, and abolish any chance I had of getting a stable career, making new friends or being successful in any field. We create an inner monologue that makes these things feel so much weightier than they really are. Rather than giving ourselves a small pat on the back for having the courage to crack that one-liner in the first place, we beat ourselves up with negative self-talk afterwards. Here are some of my inner critic's most frequent comments:

> I didn't stop talking. People probably think I love the sound of my own voice.
> I didn't talk enough. I probably came across as so rude and disinterested.
> I definitely offended her with that reply. It sounded so much more concise in my head.

On top of that, when we add emotion to the situation, sometimes a simple bit of useful feedback can turn into a personality assault for the insecure girl. I've often been scared of asking for feedback (something that's as essential as your five-a-day, when it comes to growing) in case it wasn't completely what I wanted to hear and suggested that I wasn't up to the job that I didn't think I deserved in the first place. 'I didn't enjoy this part of the book' becomes 'You are in fact the worst writer ever!'. Or, 'Ooh!

I've never seen you wear anything like that!' means 'What on earth were you thinking?'. Which, yes, seems dramatic – but sometimes receiving criticism that aligns with our own negative thoughts about ourselves can be the hardest pill to swallow. If you've ever doubted that you were deserving of a job, internship or reward and then someone else points it out, it can feel like they've taken a trip straight into your mind and confirmed your own thoughts. It's exhausting, tiring, and completely useless when it comes to making progress and taking on helpful, often necessary, advice.

Plus, in an age where unsolicited advice giving, cutting online forums and curt comments are the norm, we're so bombarded by critiques we didn't ask for that genuine feedback can get our back up.

. . . .

'I've had appearance-based comments, as well as comments about my work, and they are so hard to swallow. You assume if one person is saying it, there must be hundreds more that agree who would never say it to your face.'

CARRIE, London

. . . .

FROM THE OUTSIDE IN

Sometimes, though, these insecurities begin growing from something else. It's the magazines in the nail salon on the corner the first time we go for a manicure, dog-eared and inviting. The brazen red fonts aggressively telling us that certain body shapes are worthy of an embarrassing headline and an unforgiving front-page photograph. Research reported by *Psychology Today* estimates that we see over 5000 adverts and messages a day.[7] Those photographs that become frighteningly normal to see, that implement a 'good' and 'bad' narrative that shapes the way we see our own selves, heighten the likelihood of internal feedback from our inner critic. The first images we ever see of women's bodies are a tale of two halves – absolute scrutiny in the press, and #goals on Instagram – with the unattainable 'ideal' as accessible as an old episode of *Friends* on Comedy Central. The 2018 Girlguiding Girls' Attitudes Survey revealed that 52 per cent of girls aged 11–21 agreed with the statement: 'I sometimes feel ashamed of the way I look because I'm not like girls and women in the media.'[8] From a young age, girls commonly take part in 'makeover parties' – and although I'm perhaps being hyper-critical and a bit cynical (especially as someone who loved things like this as an eight-year-old and wanted nothing more than to be in S Club Juniors), they subliminally condition us to believe that 'before' is not the ideal, and encourage us to become aware of our appearance. As a so-called 'influencer', I'm conscious of how important it is to be mindful of how we talk about and project our appearance concerns onto others. I'm careful not to scrutinise myself online if I can; not to make excuses for doing a video without make-up or having spots, dark circles or greasy hair. It's about not apologising for the 'before' and reminding people that reality doesn't come with a flattering Instagram filter.

When it comes to your inner critic, which of the below do you find yourself worrying about?

Body image: 81% I Work: 56% I Success: 56% I Friendships: 51% I Money: 46% I Relationships: 42% I Other: 4%

Growing up, it's easy to be pigeonholed into the 'type' of person you are. 'The sporty one' or 'the clever one' or 'the pretty one'. Being given a title at such a young age can fuel your inner critic when you get older – perhaps stopping you from exploring different roles because you've taken on these assumptions and beliefs. A few years into secondary school, the mum of a friend from primary school said to me, 'Oh, you've blossomed!' and rather than saying, 'Thanks – I run a website now, have pretty good GCSEs and two years of work experience under my belt,' I felt both flattered, and like I'd achieved no more than not being the spotty eleven-year-old with eight missing teeth. I'd never been 'the pretty one', and suddenly this strange validation from a woman my mum's age was the thing that mattered most. Equally, I have friends who were regarded as 'the bright one' at school, which can so easily instil a false sense of security, and mean your inner critic is far harsher when those pigeonholed traits don't serve you as you expect when you get older.

IS IT A . . . GIRL THING?

If there's one thing we can be certain of, it's that insecurity isn't something that's gendered, ageist or selective. You can be the most confident go-getter in a room, wear both the heels and the trousers, and still be buckled by bouts of insecurity when you least expect it. However, we're constantly told there's not enough room for all of us at the table – that there can't be multiple women good at one thing or achieving greatness at any one time – with another stat from the Girlguiding Girls' Attitudes Survey 2018 showing that 67 per cent of young women aged 11–21 think women don't have the same chances as men.[9]

. . . .

'Realising there is enough room for all of us is a blessing. Especially as a woman, and a woman of colour, it is really important to open up your mind to more opportunities that society conditions you to feel are shut to you.'

NAFISAH, London

. . . .

Sometimes there's the subtler nuance where our judgement is less trusted than our male counterparts'. How many times have you been in a situation where asking a man instead of a woman has been the preferable thing to do – even if you know the same thing, or suggest the same way of handling it? Whether it's changing a light bulb, or offering a breakdown of a mind-bogglingly complicated political situation. When your capability is questioned against that of the opposite sex from a young age, sometimes it's natural to feel insecure about your ability and knowledge. There have been so many times when my boyfriend's assertions have been trusted more than mine at family dinner table political conversations (*never* a good idea in the first place). He garners more knowing head nods than I imagine a degree in politics could ever buy me – even if I've made a similar point in the past. It can often plant the seed that it's easier not to answer or offer anything at all than to risk being led to doubt your own ability.

DON'T USE THAT TONE WITH ME!

One of the things I hear most often from members of The Insecure Girls' Club is that they never know when their inner critic might start 'going off on one' (for want of a more forgiving phrase). This is definitely one of the most challenging things about dealing with your inner critic; their voice can change over time, appearing when you least expect it – or even when you're feeling vulnerable enough that you do. If you're starting a new job, chances are they'll appear (with a brazen air of authority) to criticise you, making you feel out of your depth. When you're in the changing rooms trying on something you wouldn't normally pick out, they'll quickly tell you how ridiculous you look and that 'You could never suit that!'. Sometimes it feels inescapable, noisy and stubborn – but with a bit of practice and patience, it is mutable, manageable, and it certainly doesn't have to be ever-present (or stop you wearing that brilliant new dress).

LET'S RECAP!

....

We've established that insecurity tends to spring up before we've hit adulthood – whether it's in early childhood or adolescence, or built from a series of negative memories or experiences. Those sore spots become the food of our inner critic, and it can make feedback (or, yes, sometimes real criticism) especially painful if given in relation to those subjects. Depending on what your insecurity is, the media can serve to perpetuate the idea that something about you isn't good enough, or it might be that your friends or family are making comments that seem to justify what your inner critic won't keep quiet about. Insecurity doesn't only belong to girls, but we were perhaps conditioned to feel less deserving in our younger years, and there are still stereotypes that can make us feel like the second best option compared to men.

STOP RIGHT NOW,
THANK YOU VERY MUCH

So, we've got to grips with our inner critic, but how can we take out the emotion and press pause before we start to catastrophise? And how can we feel assured that there's a seat for us at the table (even when our inner critic convinces us otherwise)? Here are some methods I've found helpful . . .

LAUGH OFF THE PAST

Aside from being an overdramatic hormone-fuelled teen worrying about a 'hairy muff', looking back, it's empowering to reclaim those moments of insecurity and embarrassment. To realise that those small, flippant words truly didn't affect my relationships, my ability to love and be loved, or the way I view myself today. With hindsight, I can now enjoy a moment of hair-flipping sass when I think of all those silly comments that made me feel 'less than'. And, though it's disproportionately teenage girls who have to contend with that kind of pressure, when it comes to looking back to past mistakes, nasty comments and those itches that have your toes curling every time you revisit memory lane, know that they don't define you. They won't stop you growing, progressing or doing brilliant things – and whether you've got hair 'down there' or not will never make a difference. It's desperately hard at the time to laugh it off – I remember crying into an ex-boyfriend's voicemail when he dumped me over Myspace (I know) and thinking it would follow me around for years to come, but guess what: it didn't! I always ask myself, 'Will this still be such a big deal in a year's time?'. Chances are, it won't. If you can see the situation happening to a character in your favourite sitcom, it's probably just a minute detail in the bigger picture and will only be a small imprint in the big ol' fabric of your life.

**Can you describe a mistake in your past
that you've learnt from?**

'I let my insecurities get the better of me, leading me to
depression. I learnt that believing in myself can take me
further than any external validation.'   *Sevi, London*

'UNHOOK' FROM PRAISE AND CRITICISM

As much as I encourage silencing the negative back-chat we
give ourselves, sometimes we can harness these voices as
a means for good, a driving force to help us do better and
recognise our goals. A little like how jealousy can shine a
light on the things you want to achieve for yourself, your
inner critic can be flipped upside down, revealing something good about you – rather than a weakness.

One thing I've learnt over the last few years, after a very
generous introduction from my friend Charlotte, is the
power of 'unhooking' from praise and criticism. Wonder
woman Tara Mohr, the expert in tackling our inner critic,
explains how to manage both praise and criticism in a way
that makes us realise that neither is personal on any level –
and furthermore that they can be as useful or disposable
as we want them to be. In her book *Playing Big*, she covers
how our inner critic 'has no interest in actual evidence',

suggesting most of the time it's just not true.[10] In short, our 'most distinctive' work or actions will always get a reaction – but the feedback we receive tells us more about the person giving it than us. My favourite tip of Tara's is: 'Look up one of your favourite books on Amazon. Read a five-star review. Then read a one-star review. Notice the diversity of reactions. This is a great way to see that even incredible work doesn't earn universal praise.'[11]

IDENTIFY THE OUTSIDE ELEMENTS

If there are people in your life who feed into this negative self-talk and mirror what your inner critic is saying to you, it's worth asking why you allow them into your life. If it's a parent or someone who's part of your everyday life (who it's not possible to 'cut out'), maybe it's time for a conversation about how they're making you feel. The thing about your inner critic is that they're in your head. But when those negative comments leak into an external narrative, it's important to re-evaluate who is truly worthy of your company and makes you feel better about yourself, rather than worse. Sometimes people might say these things to protect you, but if it's starting to shape a negative opinion of yourself, you must let that person know how you feel. The conversation doesn't have to be approached with aggression or upset, but perhaps with something along the lines of: 'I notice you keep bringing up X, which isn't making me feel very good', or, 'I'd rather we didn't keep talking about X as it's making me feel a bit rubbish.' These conversations can be really uncomfortable and difficult (trust me, I know), but often we forego them to keep everyone else happy – without checking that we are happy ourselves. Anyone that has your best interests at heart should understand where you're coming from, and can hopefully shift the narrative for the better.

REMEMBER, WE'RE ALL IN THE SAME BOAT

I vividly remember first being asked to meet a handful of editors when this book you're holding(!) was little more than a twinkle in my eye. Despite feeling a total blur of undeserved excitement, it was the textbook 'big scary meeting' that required about four toilet trips beforehand (which naturally means I can direct you to some of the best free loos in London), some emergency texts from friends (kindly reminding me that if things got *really bad*, Imodium is always brilliant), and a quick pit stop for some peppermint tea (because what else do you do in this situation?). But once we'd all sat down, a feeling of calm swept over me. We are all feeling these things. One of the women opened up about how she'd been feeling nervous too, and then it became apparent that we all had these things going on – the playing field was pretty level. It dawned on me that perhaps we'd all run for a train that morning, spilt some cereal down our new Zara top, had become a bit sweaty and then worried things wouldn't go well in the meeting. It made me realise how easy it is to assume you're the only person in the room feeling incapable and out of your depth. But take away the mystery with some small talk, and you'll be surprised to find that more often than not, you're not the only one feeling like that. Whoever we are, our inner critic confronts us all at some point, and although its comments might be masked as unwelcome negative talk from ourselves, it's actually something quite separate from us that catches us all off guard when we need it least.

MAKE YOUR INNER CRITIC A CHARACTER . . .

Obviously, there's a big difference between the kinds of things we say to ourselves, and what we should say and how that can be useful. Typically, the 'super-ego' voice in our head is hyperbolic, cruel and inaccurate. Imagine your inner critic personified and looking like an evil Bond villain (or angry chauvinist driver) with a deep furrowed brow and cackling laugh. Give it a name if you like, and write down the things that your inner critic says to you. I did this and was surprised at how quickly I could recognise how ridiculous, hurtful and plain unhelpful these things really are – and that if it was a real person in the street talking to me like this, I'd never allow myself to be spoken to in that way, nor would I ever speak to anyone else like that either.

**What do you do if you realise you're
being unkind to yourself?**

'I berate myself through negative thought, so I try to catch
myself by doing a task I have been meaning to do. Feeling
productive is usually the first step out of an insecure head-
space for me.'   *Lucy, London*

. . . AND TALK BACK TO IT!

If you struggle to separate yourself from your inner critic,
then that's when you need to work on silencing it, or
making it 'work' for you. Unpick the drama from what the
inner critic is saying and try to identify whether there is
anything of use in it.

. . . .

'I've done a lot of work on trying to understand the
human brain, and how a lot of our thoughts are stories. Repeating patterns in our brain, we can change
those stories and unpick them. Every time I catch
myself doing it, I'm like, "Where is the evidence?! Oh,
another bullshit story I'm telling myself . . ." NEXT.'
                                    CHARLOTTE, Lincoln

. . . .

For example, instead of saying to yourself, 'Oh my goodness, you're a nightmare to listen to', switch it up and say, 'I might talk a lot, but I have lots of interesting things to share.' It's so important to remember that your inner critic isn't an accurate reflection of who you are or how you're behaving. It's there to protect you if it recognises scary or intimidating situations, but often it ends up putting you off and making you feel incapable. Knowing when to stop it in its tracks, pinch its lips shut and shake it off is the first stepping stone to self-confidence.

What we say *vs* what we should say

God, you're such an idiot! Why do you always put your foot in it?
Good on you for braving that! No one else was speaking up!

She's doing so much better than you are.
You're both at different stages, and yes she's doing well – but look how much you've achieved!

You don't deserve that job/result/promotion.
YES, GIRL, YES! Although it was a surprise, you worked so hard: you definitely earned it!

Also, check in with those around you who know you as well as you know yourself. When Lauren, a London-based member of The Insecure Girls' Club, feels this way, she looks outwards: 'I tend to throw myself into family and friends as they act as a mirror – if they like me, then maybe I'm not that bad!'. It can be hard to see the bigger picture when you're in the throes of an insecure blip; aiming to be around people who love and care for you is invaluable when it comes to getting a fresh perspective.

Africa Brooke
mindset coach and speaker

After stumbling across Africa on Instagram and inhaling all of her BCW (big caption wisdom) on everything from friendships and garnering self-belief to tackling your inner critic, I knew I had to speak to her. Online (and off) she discusses in depth and with honesty everything from imposter syndrome to money management and assuming failure in a way that'll have you feeling like you can take on the world.

Africa, your career and page (@africabrooke) cover all areas of self-development – how did you start talking about this, and how did it all begin?
It all began in 2016 when I finally got sober after many failed attempts at removing alcohol from my life. Due to shame and cultural conditioning, I didn't seek professional help or recovery groups offline. I went online to find a community I couldn't seem to access in my day-to-day life – and this is how the platform I have today was built. Although I battled heavily with my inner critic at the start of my journey – 'you will never be able to stay sober', 'are you sure you should be sharing so much online?' – I persevered and gave myself

permission to rewrite my narrative and inspire others to do the same.

You speak a lot about self-sabotage, which comes hand in hand with your inner critic. How do you stop yourself from being unkind to yourself?
I do this by not heavily identifying with my thoughts. Meaning, I have come to the point of realising that I AM NOT MY THOUGHTS, and I don't have to respond to or action every negative thought that comes into my mind. This takes compassion, patience and PRACTICE. I allow myself to feel whatever needs to be felt, be it anger, sadness, resentment, jealousy, envy, etc. Then I question where it's coming from and accept it for what it is at the time. Of course, this might sound simplistic – but the 'simplest' things are always the most powerful once practised with intention.

I think one thing that fuels our inner critic so much is the fear of being disliked, which is exhausting. It can make us forget who we are in our own heads. Have you felt like this, and how have you managed to step away from it?
I have definitely felt like this! And I too believe that a lot of the fear we feel is tied to wanting acceptance of some sort. I have something in my toolkit called a Proof List. For example, when I have my inner critic berating me for 'not doing enough', I'll write out a list of all the things I've accomplished in that week, month or year as actual proof that this voice has no idea what it's talking about. I'll then read each one out loud and place the list somewhere visible. It's a good method to detach from the unhelpful opinions that bombard us each and every waking day.

What are your top three tips for hushing your inner critic?

- Collecting actual proof that the inner critic is wrong (journal a list or get feedback from trusted pals).
- Understanding that YOU ARE NOT YOUR THOUGHTS ('I am not my thoughts' is a great mantra).
- Feeling the doubt and fear yet taking action anyway! (CAUTION: this one is powerful!)

Finally, you're a fountain of knowledge when it comes to looking after ourselves – do you have any words of compassion or mantras for members of The Insecure Girls' Club to add to their repertoire?

THE MIND ISN'T ALWAYS ON YOUR SIDE! (Remember this because it can change everything.) It's worth knowing that the mind is just doing its best to protect you from perceived pain, even when it's being a meanie. Its job is to keep you comfortable, safe and basically alive, but it still gets it very wrong sometimes. Although it's impossible to completely get rid of negative thoughts, it is very much possible to work with them so that they don't have so much power over your life and every decision you make. And the best way to start training this muscle is to make a commitment to not believe or action *everything* the mind tells you.

ASK – WHO ARE YOU COMPETING WITH?

Is your inner critic fuelling a competitiveness which is making you feel 'less than' when it comes to weighing up what you're doing, compared with others? If so, it might be time to check in with yourself – where you are compared with your own goals and expectations. Try to recognise that this isn't a race, and that sometimes stepping back to refuel is the best thing.

If you're feeling a little lost with where to begin when it comes to checking in with yourself and working out what it is you want (instead of what you keep seeing online), here are three ways to reclaim that focus:
- Create a vision board. This is a bit like a mood board or scrapbook page, except it's solely centred on you. Grab a piece of card or a cork-board and start pinning, sticking or taping on cut-outs from magazines or newspapers, featuring words or images that spring out at you, or get yourself onto Pinterest (or even collections on Instagram) and start getting pin happy. Putting everything in one place can really show where your inspiration lies (or even the things you didn't realise were important to you), prompting and pointing

you in the right direction. Plus, who doesn't love a bit of an *Art Attack* moment?

- Take a break. Sometimes stepping away from competitiveness means taking a break from the source of the competition. Are you sitting on Facebook and feeling out of your depth? Is there a group of friends who don't make you feel great? Spend a few days without social media and do something after work or school that *you* enjoy, something that'll make you feel capable and good about yourself. Take a dance class, schedule in a cuppa with your bestie, practise some writing – you could even take a spin on Duolingo and get practising that new language you've been putting off. Do something that'll make you feel 'more than', and not less.

- Take it step by step. If you're setting painfully high expectations for yourself that you're finding you can't fulfil or manage, then strip things back a bit. Take each day at a time, and maybe create smaller, more achievable steps to getting where you want. For example, if you've always dreamt of opening a bakery but year after year realise you still haven't had the grand opening, then begin smaller. Start an Instagram account for your baking – share your page with those closest to you and see where it leads. Make things achievable so that the bigger goals don't feel so far off.

CLAIM THAT TIME BACK

Finally, if we think about the time we spend second-guessing our own judgements and actions, could it be spent doing something a lot more positive and productive? Instead of listing everything you feel you're not great at, look at creating small daily affirmations and little cards to pep you up for the day ahead.

. . . .

'I went through a stage where I was being so unkind to myself that I'd write myself little notes of encouragement, and stick them around my room where I'd see them, as a way to remind myself of my good qualities.'

MOLLY, Kent

. . . .

Sometimes it takes pointing out the good to silence the bad. Your affirmations can be general statements, or a list of things you've proved you're capable of.

Here are a handful of my favourite Instagram accounts for positive affirmations:

- @alifemoreinspired – creative coach Nicola shares inspiring and uplifting affirmations for adults and children, and a thirty-four-card pack for daily pick-me-ups.
- @britandco – beautifully illustrated daily affirmations and power quotes for on-the-go 'I got this'.
- @oh_squirrel – picture-perfect motivational posters and postcards (the ultimate gift to self).
- @growing.basil – tattoo artist and illustrator Fiona sells double-sided affirmation cards and posts gorgeous Instagrams for inspired scrolling.
- @iamstevienelson – photographer and actress Stevie sells her pack of pocket mantras, which she initially painted as a pick-me-up and realised it was something we could all do with.

Takeaway pick-me-ups for hushing your inner critic, from The Insecure Girls' Club

- Laugh at the past – reclaim moments of insecurity and embarrassment because they don't define you going forwards.
- Listen to Tara Mohr – know that your inner critic has 'no interest in actual evidence', so try to shake off the silliness when it strikes.
- Found that someone is starting to affirm the negative things you say to yourself? Pull them up and have a gentle word – you don't need to take it from all angles!
- Know that you're never alone in feeling like this – everyone has had to deal with this chatter at some point, even the people you admire the most.
- Personify your inner critic, if you can – preferably as the ultimate movie baddie – so you can realise how you truly don't need their input.
- Have a think – would you talk to someone you love as unkindly as you talk to yourself? If you wouldn't, then nip it in the bud straight away.
- Finally, if you fancy it, whip out some affirmation cards and get spiritual every morning – because you are very much worth it.

2

'I'm not as good as her': tackling comparison and the art of doing it differently

Just because you're doing it differently,
doesn't mean you're doing it wrong

I remember when I first stumbled across a perfectly inked calligraphy drawing of the saying 'comparison is the thief of joy' on Pinterest. Pinned alongside a 'Dream big. Laugh lots.' quote, strangely it was the Theodore Roosevelt number that truly struck a chord with me. This guy *gets* it, I thought to myself – what a hero! Before, naturally, I shared it, I scribbled it everywhere, and reminded myself of it daily whenever I felt the twinge of a wobble around the corner. Ironically, this was long before Instagram became my most used social media app (in fact, before it even existed). In a way, pinning then what is now one of the most popular mantras when it comes to comparison was the first tool in my mental arsenal for tackling it – and what became a long stretch of navigating this ongoing insecurity.

Comparison isn't a new thing. It existed before Instagram

was even a twinkle in Kevin Systrom and Mike Krieger's eyes (the founders of your favourite app, in case you aren't on first-name terms). A study from two French universities suggested that women are unconsciously conditioned to social comparison, finding evidence that subliminal exposure to the 'thin ideal' (in this case, 'media images of ultra-thin women') increased body appearance anxiety in women, strongly affecting their self-evaluations. So it's something we don't even necessarily realise we're doing.[12]

What triggers comparison for you?

'I work in academia, so I constantly feel like I'm not as smart as my colleagues. I feel like Elle Woods in that scene where she goes to her first lecture and is completely overwhelmed.'   *Jasmine, London*

I remember there was a 'Learning to Learn' club in secondary school, which essentially aimed to improve high-achieving students' capabilities and reward them with things like trips to Thorpe Park (the peak theme-park destination of teenage cool) and vouchers for WHSmith. Not being invited to be part of the club was one of the first times I felt comparison. I felt the 'Oh *shit*, I'm not smart enough to be rewarded' pang, and the little green-eyed monster on my shoulder that meant I was able to quickly dismiss any of my own achievements, instead focusing on how much better everyone around me was, and how much smarter everyone else *had* to be.

And that's another thing – comparison and jealousy run hand in hand. This emotion has the power to make everyone seem like they're having a way better time than you are, that they're better than you and probably have what you want too. It feels like the least admirable thing to admit to, even if you're completely swimming in it. There's an episode of *Sabrina the Teenage Witch* where she has to walk around school in sunglasses because her jealousy of her best friend is so bad her eyes leak green, but we know the truth of Sabrina's words when she says, 'If everyone else has great stuff, it doesn't take away all of the wonderful things that I have.' Who'd have thought one of my most poignant teenage lessons would come from a teenage witch?

COMPARISON ON SOCIAL MEDIA

If comparison is based on an innate need to be liked and accepted, the way social media works validates those feelings tenfold. Every time a little heart appears on the bottom right-hand corner of our screen, it's the validation we so crave, and that hit of recognition (in the form of dopamine, also known as the feel-good hormone) makes us feel liked. It's clear that comparison is more regularly induced and exacerbated by social media. Because even if 'in real life' we are satisfied, loved and respected, the need to be approved online can sometimes feel more important.

We can seek approval from a stranger across the world more than we look to the real nurtured relationships we have sitting right in front of us – how strange is that?

Sometimes it feels like old friends, new friends, celebrities, colleagues, bloggers, Instagrammers and everyone in between are auditioning for a lead role in this year's comparison vision board. The worst thing is, there are no parameters to enforce rational comparison on social media. You can compare your gym activity to someone who's promoting a fitness DVD and 'ten-minute healthy meal' cookbook, or your skin to someone who has the time and money for four facials a week and a bathroom cupboard with more lotions and potions than Lloyds Pharmacy. It's the hollowness of seeing everyone else out and about when you're at home being asked if you're still watching by Netflix, even when the people who are out are envying you being inside. It's a never-ending chase-your-tail circle that sometimes feels like there's always a more fun and more exciting option.

Who do you compare yourself to the most?

Friends: 52% | Celebrities/Influencers: 26% | Colleagues: 13% | Other: 6% | Family: 2% | Nobody: 1%

And in that same breath, those strangers are the people we often end up comparing ourselves to the most. We're so intent on looking at what @stylishsally567 in Paris is wearing that we forget the clothes we have in our own ward-robes. What holiday @harrietholiday111 is taking and how much better that is than our week off in July will be. Despite knowing nothing about these people's personal lives, or their existences beyond an edited image online, we're subliminally competing and comparing them with our own reality, making the self-inflicted pressure to always be 'better' inescapable.

On top of that, nowadays not only are we compar-ing pictures of designer outfits and luxury five-star honeymoon-worthy holidays, but sometimes we're engag-ing in intellectual comparison too: how articulate we are online about what's going on in the world, how great an activist we can be, and how 'woke' we are. It's progressive and amazing that social media content creators and influ-encers are encouraged to speak about these things – but sometimes the pressure of always getting it right ('con-science comparison', as I like to call it), comparing our-selves to others who are doing it better and being 'cleverer', leaves little room for getting there ourselves and cultivat-ing our own stances. It doesn't matter if we don't always understand the news, haven't read the whole Booker prize shortlist, or can't always keep up in a lecture. Our intellect comes in many shapes and forms – and not knowing it all in one place leaves room for you to be brilliant in another.

. . . .

'I'll get to things when I'm good and ready. (Insert sarcastic eye roll.) But seriously, it's hard not to compare myself to everyone and say, "Oh shit, I'm behind."'

RANDI, California

. . . .

Comparison creeps up on us in real life too. Whether it's the girl sweeping the board with A*s or your friend at the office who's a creative genius, comparison is inescapable. After years of undervaluing my achievements, thinking I had accomplished less because I wasn't matching up to people I didn't know (or worse, people I did), I became determined to change my mindset towards one of the biggest triggers of insecurity we just can't seem to shake.

'I SHOULD HAVE DONE [INSERT MILESTONE HERE] BY NOW!'

Has there been a time when someone else has done something and you've thought, 'I should be doing that'?

'Seeing people I went to school with buying a house or getting married made me feel like a failure. Especially on social media, where everything is presented as the best life.'   *Anon*

One easy metric for comparison IRL is age – looking around at people younger than you and wondering why you haven't quite achieved everything in your years that they have in theirs. Age can so easily feel like the simplest way of justifying comparison – and it works both ways too. Getting to a certain age and feeling like you should have ticked certain boxes – be it owning a house or getting married – or looking back at points in your life when you 'should' have done something because the next person did, or society expected it of you.

. . . .

'A close friend of mine, who is the same age, graduated a year later than me. By the time she got her degree she had already been offered an amazing job in her dream field. I know that before this she was just as scared as I was of the future; she was still scared and insecure. But from the outside, it seemed to me that she was thriving – working in the industry she wanted to, enjoying life and her job.'

MORGANE, France

. . . .

From the outside, it's so easy to perceive achievements and 'success' as linear, and I think we've all been there when we've felt 'behind' – be it at work, in our studies or personal milestones.

It can also feel incredibly difficult when other people seemingly 'get lucky' and land on their feet. Morgane continues: 'I know [my friend] worked hard, but I felt like in comparison I was failing. From where I stood, everything had happened to her easily. I worked just as hard as her and had been trying for longer, so why couldn't I be successful?' It can be hard to accept someone excelling or getting further along on their journey when you know you've put in just as much legwork. But in reality, the idea of someone 'excelling' or 'getting ahead' is only valid if life is a race – and as we said earlier, it's really not. Owning your own timeline and trusting that your hard work will pay off is key here – and just because someone got somewhere first, doesn't mean you won't get there at all. Plus, being able to celebrate another's success won't ever make *you* less successful – it'll just help you feel a lot better about it in the short term, because celebrating always feels better than wallowing in disappointment or envy.

. . . .

'I think when someone around your age is doing something you'd love to do it can bring up feelings of comparison. It can feel a bit like someone else's success is an indicator of your own failure: particularly as you get older and it feels more and more like your lot in life is set in stone. The truth is that it isn't. Things can always change and there's no rush to success. I work in Parliament, and before I did I was interested in being an MP. Inspired by Alexandria Ocasio-Cortez and Mhairi Black, I aspired to become a young politician. Having worked for an MP I can see why the average age is fifty – the financial insecurity surrounding campaigning, the pressure, the unsociable working hours, the difficulty of balancing it with raising a family. All of these things, which need to be combatted, make me think that if I want to be an MP it's really OK, if not beneficial, to take my time and to gain more life experience before going down that route.'

GENEVIEVE, London

. . . .

For years after I dropped out of university, I remember seeing Facebook photos of mortarboard hats raining from the sky, champagne emoji bottles popping and '2:1, GUYS!' statuses – all making me wonder if I'd totally done the wrong thing by leaving, when 'this' was the time I was 'meant' to be graduating. It felt like my pathway through the final years of full-time education hadn't been straight and narrow, but sideways and really quite zig-zagged. Rather than collecting my results and deciding which restaurant I wanted to be taken to for dinner to celebrate, I was hidden away in a dark and dingy fashion cupboard attempting to gain work experience. At the time it felt like a poor decision on my part. I'd bypassed a degree for fashion returns and travel expenses – but looking back with the power of hindsight, I should have realised that just because you haven't taken the same path as someone else, it doesn't mean the things you want to achieve won't happen for you. Success isn't linear, and it truly looks different for everyone.

NO TWO GOALS ARE THE SAME

Said in my favourite American powerhouse TED talk voice, of course. One thing that always helps me out of a comparison rut is remembering that not everyone's goals are the same. Online, it can sometimes feel like there is one textbook definition of a #GirlBoss and one only. Google defines it as: 'A confident, capable woman who pursues her own ambitions instead of working for others or otherwise settling in life.' Which is all well and good – but what about the rest of us? The ones who work for huge companies in big teams and are perfectly happy not leading them? The ones who are self-employed but sometimes feel so shrouded by the overwhelming competitiveness and expectation of being a #GirlBoss that they forget why they started?

. . . .

'One of the biggest game changers for me was purposefully using the word "we" more when working as a team and leaving the word "I" out of things as much as possible. It's such an obvious thing, but even if I have been working on something fairly independently, I now consciously use the word "we" to include the whole team. That way, there's no room for competitiveness, and everyone works together and feels proud of everyone's contributions. I found it to be a really good tactic for my own mindset.'

LAUREN, Rutland

. . . .

Sometimes we don't even realise we have a 'goal', because we've never looked at it that way. For some people just getting through the day is more than enough, and that's perfect. Have a proper think about what your goals look like to you – and use them as your road map. You can look out of the window at other people you pass on the road, but being able to look, accept and keep on trucking is crucial. We are going to have to see other people's successes in life no matter how hard we try, but knowing how not to let them faze us is the key to staying on track.

Not motivated by money? Fine! Don't fancy managing a team of ten and holding boardroom meetings? No problem! As long as you're doing something that makes you happy (most of the time, anyway), then keep on kicking. I'll watch people tackle endless boot-camp-style personal training sessions and think, 'Shit, should I be doing that? Have I been super unproductive today?' when it simply isn't something that – as Marie Kondo would say – sparks joy for me. Not everyone has to strive for a blockbuster film deal, a sell-out arena tour and a million followers on Instagram – and how boring would it be if we all did?

THE DIFFERENT MEANINGS
OF HARD WORK

For years, one of the biggest markers of comparison for me was the way in which I worked. As a freelancer I create my own working hours, am fully in charge of self-motivation, meeting deadlines and making sure things are getting ticked off – be that emails, accounts, admin or, of course, the whole creative side. Although most of the time I can recognise that being my own boss is an enormous privilege, looking at other small business owners (or in fact anyone who's working), it's amazing to see the discrepancy in different people's definitions of 'busy' and 'hard-working'.

For me, being 'hard-working' means having a steady flow of work, making sure it's completed on time to the best of my ability, and being able to finish each day at a reasonable hour. I remember once seeing someone on Twitter talk about how they were still up working at 3 a.m., and rather than think, 'God, shouldn't she be getting some sleep?' my reaction was, 'Oh God, should I be working like that?'

After reading Rebecca Holman's book *Beta: Quiet Girls Can Run the World*,[13] I realised there was so much power in asserting the different ways we, as women, can work. It showed me that being an 'alpha' working woman who juggles four businesses, three children, and goes on holiday every weekend needn't be the thing that defines success for me. Our culture praises women who work themselves to the bone as the most hard-working and the best at their jobs, and for so long this made me think that to be great at my career, that's what I had to do.

But doing well isn't necessarily working weekends or late into the night. It's about getting things done, in a reasonable time, at a pace that complements your life. How many times have you felt pressure to stay later at work just because a few 'hard-working' people were carrying on? Rather than feeling guilty, did you think that perhaps they simply weren't as efficient at their work, or using their time as productively? Just because you work differently, doesn't mean you need to overcompensate to prove it. Working differently doesn't mean you're not working at all.

THE (FALSE) BRILLIANCE OF BEING BUSY

The same goes for being 'busy'. Oh, that word. The word we love to hate. The word that can feel like the true marker of being cool and 'in demand' and something we all crave to be, painting a picture of a chic woman walking out of a coffee shop with a pink neon sign, designer handbag in tow and off to a glamorous meeting.

I'd often see Instagram captions about how 'busy' people's lives were, and how much they had coming up(!) as I sat at home fumbling together a blog post in two-day-old pyjamas, with a lone Coco Pop glued to the collar. The reality of my 'busy' was very different. For me it was not forgetting to reply to friends' WhatsApp messages because I'd been juggling an overflowing inbox. Remembering to do a budget food shop (no plastic bags) because otherwise I'd overspend in M&S on the way home again. Not forgetting the vet appointment and not letting the vegetables in the fridge go mushy and stick to the bottom. Like success, the definition of 'busy' is messy, complex, and far less polished than we tend to give it credit for.

'BUT WHY ME?' – TACKLING
IMPOSTER SYNDROME

Where comparison and success circulate, in steps our friend 'imposter syndrome': when you feel like you don't deserve to be where you are, or that your success is unearned. A nationwide study of 3000 adults found that two thirds of women in the UK suffer from imposter syndrome at work[14] – so if this sounds familiar to you, you're not alone.

In my career, I can think of endless occasions when I've walked into an event, looked around with pure unadulterated fear, and then turned to walk out again. I remember arriving at a dinner on the roof of a private members' club (where, naturally, I was very much not a member), clocking lots of people who would never recognise me, and being poached by the lady who had invited me, then sitting nervously all evening, legs jiggling, texting 'HELP, I DON'T KNOW WHAT TO SAY' to my mum from under the table.

Imposter syndrome for me is being surrounded by circles of people with official job titles and crystal-clear skill sets, leaving me wondering what I'm doing there and what *my* role is. The inner mutterings of 'Why am I here?', 'Who invited *me*?!' and '*Oh my god if someone asks why I'm here I'll have no idea what to tell them because I HAVE NO IDEA EITHER*'. The times I've wanted to say to a brand, 'But why would you want to work with me?' before having to give myself a stern talking to and avoid genuinely putting them off working with me. It's the continued self-critique that gets in the way of new opportunities and allowing others to believe in you – because, ultimately, you don't believe in yourself.

. . . .

'I felt like I was there [in my first graduate job] as the result of serendipitous luck and one day they would realise I wasn't cut out for the job. The firsts didn't stop coming. In hindsight, they were a sign that my boss trusted me. But inside, it felt like the more things I didn't know how to do, the more times I had to pretend I was OK and "can so handle this". Once I knew about it [imposter syndrome], I could understand all the sleepless nights I'd had before presentations, the constant chorus of self-criticism, my tendency to explain away my success, and the ongoing fear of being exposed. The next time I got THE FEAR that I'd be unmasked as a fraud, I could name it for what it was – imposter syndrome.'

LOUISE, Birmingham

. . . .

All of these feelings continue to feel familiar to so many of us, and it's imperative to remind ourselves about the little wins that will help our confidence in our capabilities to grow and be able to recognise our value. Learn to start saying, '*This* is why I was chosen,' and, 'Wow, I've worked hard to get here,' instead of feeling fraudulent and ready to be 'found out'. We all have the right to a good shot at something, and every time I feel like I'm out of my depth, underqualified or being fraudulent, I remind myself of that.

LET'S RECAP!

. . . .

So, we've had a big old chat about comparison – from its roots in real life to how it manifests online when we find ourselves scrolling on autopilot, and the jealousy that can rear its head after too much looking sideways and not enough self-appreciation. From looking at focusing on our own goals, how being busy and hard-working is different for everyone (and can have different definitions depending on who you are), and why imposter syndrome is something best left outside the workplace (alongside sneaky under-the-desk scrolling. Ahem).

STOP RIGHT NOW, THANK YOU VERY MUCH

So what's next in beating the chorus of comparison? How do we start appreciating ourselves as much as we do others online, how can we use social media to make ourselves feel good, and how can we be a #GirlBoss without changing anything?

USING SOCIAL MEDIA RIGHT

One of the first steps to cutting out comparison is knowing how to recognise when you're not spending your time wisely online. When the minutes creep into hours, and the time you could have spent doing something you truly love (or finally starting *Game of Thrones*) has whittled away into broken minutes that often leave you feeling worse than before you started (and still with no idea who the Mother of Dragons is).

What do you do when you recognise you've spent too much time online?

Switch off: 50% | Keep scrolling: 38% | Other: 9% | None of the above: 4%

It's easy to say 'stop scrolling', but it's not so easy to do – especially if you have to use apps like Instagram for work. Here are some ideas for new habits that make scrolling a more pleasant experience if you can't go cold turkey straight away:

- Use the 'mute' button. Quiet the noise of people who get your goat, who you compare yourself to, or who make you feel 'less than' (this is particularly useful if you don't want to 'unfollow' someone – out of guilt or 'the politics' around it, and the tension that this sometimes brings).
- Shift your perspective. If you find yourself diving deep into the feeds and highlights of other people,

start looking at your own Instagram in that way too. Use it as a record for all your own personal wins and happy memories, and a reminder of everything you've done and achieved.

- Curate, curate, curate! Create a feed that reflects your own interests, and the things that make you feel inspired and fulfilled. This is so much more important than following big brands, or celebrities who make you feel pressured, unsuccessful or behind in life. To quote Russell Brand, 'Don't you generate enough negativity in your own consciousness without finding external systems to replicate it?'[15] Deep, but true!

- Download a mobile usage-tracking app like Moment. Sometimes simply being aware of the time you're wasting scrolling and arguably 'self-sabotaging' can be a little push to distance yourself from social media and get back into your own lane. One of the truest things I've ever read – in Daisy Buchanan's *How to Be a Grown-Up* – is: 'You're capable of amazing things, but you might miss them if you don't stop comparing yourself with other people and their achievements.'[16]

Lucy Sheridan
comparison coach

With all the scope there is for comparing ourselves, there's an opportunity for wonderful women like Lucy Sheridan to create platforms and arenas to ease people out of social media comparison. If you're ever in need of a pick-me-up online, or a nudge out of a comparison trap, Lucy is your lady. Offering inspiring tips, tangible advice and endless knowledge, she's a breath of fresh air when it comes to tackling comparison.

Lucy, you're the world's first and only comparison coach, which is mega! Can you tell us how it all began?
Comparison for me has been 'teach what we need to learn', and it's something that has followed me around a lot. It was interesting because I didn't realise that so much of my purpose would be so tied up in something that I was trying to run away from. Having gone to a school reunion I started comparing myself to different people all the time. I'd explored self-development and was also doing a life-coaching course (just like you would do an embroidery course on the side). It was very much a passion project, where I wanted to understand a bit more about myself.

I had a very odd experience where I heard [my inner] voice when I was in a meeting, which said, 'I won't let you pick the time, but I'll give you what you want.' I thought, 'Whoa, this is strange,' but I took it as a real call to take a leap of faith. I resigned the next day, but thought, 'I'll go self-employed, and on the side I'll see if I can get in some coaching clients.' A journalist who was doing a piece on overthinking approached me on Twitter, and during the conversation I just spoke the phrase 'comparison coaching'. So I thought I'd give myself ninety days on this and see if it took off. And whilst it sounds clichéd to say that the rest is history, that was definitely the beginning.

Comparison is something that we find ourselves talking about more and more. If we're in an office or even if it's your friend at school, why do you think that we do it?
I think firstly, by talking about it more, the taboo is dissolving around it. It's almost built into our DNA: 'Thou shalt not covet' is one of the Ten Commandments, and 'keeping up with the Joneses' was an expression developed in the nineteenth century, and from 1913–1938 turned into a cartoon strip about fighting for status. But I think that the main reason why we do it is because we become disconnected from ourselves, and somewhere along the line we start to put other people's opinions ahead of ours, and we start to put other people's definitions of success in front of or instead of our own. We do it because we get given so many cues, directions, advice and instructions on what it is we should be doing and what we should be experiencing, and if you don't have that strongly rooted feeling of being in your life and connecting with your choices, it's so easy to be spinning around like a moon around a planet.

Why do you think we compare ourselves to people who have completely different paths, goals and experiences?
It's funny, isn't it, because confidence is sexy, so we're attracted to that. I think that can trigger our comparison, because regardless of what they're confident about, it's the idea that they're in alignment and going towards their purpose that shows a fulfilment, and we're like a moth to a flame. My work is about guiding people through self-focus and self-confidence and ultimately self-worth. But I think that why we do it is because we haven't given ourselves permission to give ourselves what we want. A lot of our goals, or what we think motivates us, are inherited. So: 'my dad wanted this', or 'this has always run in our family', or 'everyone in our town does this', or 'my friend got me into this'. Comparison can really thrive when we don't check the signposting.

So many of us use age as a barometer of success and what we 'should' be doing. Is there a better way of looking at it than 'I should have done that by this age'?
I saw a video on Facebook a few years ago, and it used the analogy of time zones. It said that nobody accuses New York of being behind Barcelona because New York wakes up six hours later; they're just in different time zones. Ultimately time zones are all completely unique to us.

It's really making sure that you don't become obsessed with these things, and that you throw your weight and support behind people who are doing the things that you want to do. So if you're feeling uncomfortable or feeling like time is running out, that's bullshit.

Do you have three quick tips to battle comparison day to day?

The first one is that if you can feel it coming up, get offline and do some big belly breathing.

Secondly, flood your feed and your senses with things that light you up and you want to do. So, for example, if you start your day with three–five gratitudes, it immediately allows the day to rise up and meet you – and everything else will just come onto your plate as the day goes on, but you're still robust in yourself.

One thing I do when I'm feeling like this is to take my right hand and place it onto my pulse, and feel my actual life energy running under the tips of my fingers – if you've ever doubted how special you are then that's the one – and then with the other hand I'll rub my heart and say, 'You're all right, kid, you're all right.' It's this tremendously soothing experience, and I find that really, really centring.

Lastly, do you have a mantra or a few words of compassion that you can give to members of The Insecure Girls' Club?

Every day, and in every way, in expected and unexpected ways, my life is working out for me.

START THE DAY DIFFERENTLY

One of the tips I frequently hear that is always, always true is to start the day without looking at your phone for the first hour (or two, if you're brave). I know. Hear me out. This is not because it's not essential to see which new cute cat GIFs have surfaced online during your slumber, but because it's important to start your day without knowing how everybody else started theirs. Imagine a morning when you feel accomplished from getting up after one snooze (and not ten) instead of defeated because you didn't pack in a 6 a.m. legs, bums and tums class. Praise yourself for the things that you know you did well, as opposed to beating yourself up for the things you were never going to do in the first place. Being comfortable on your own without distractions (digital or otherwise) can be useful for muting comparison too, and becoming happier with yourself.

'I'm not as good as her'

. . . .

'If I'm on the tram to work, rather than being a slave to my phone like all the other commuters, I take notice of my fellow passengers, the passing views of North Manchester, the kindness of the passenger offering up their seat to the young mum. Being mindful of the world around me helps me to realise there is more to life than how many likes you get on Instagram, or what so-and-so had for breakfast.'

LUCY, Manchester

. . . .

Allow time to be solo, enjoy your own company, and discover who you want to be without trying to be an amalgamation of others, or a version of somebody you saw online.

What is it you enjoy doing offline, in your spare time? Here are some suggestions if you're stuck for ideas:
- Get baking! Pull out a dusty recipe book that's been neglected and try something new.
- Go swimming in your local lido (this always makes me feel very sophisticated).

- Do a bit of drawing at home – or reignite a creative activity you used to do. I love a bit of a doodle when I'm watching TV.
- See if there are any exhibitions in town that you fancy – there are so many small free ones that will leave you feeling cultured. Every day is a school day!
- Go vintage shopping! I love a rummage around a charity shop, and it means I don't have to go too far from home.
- If you have to do a mundane task like tidying or sorting, put together some Spotify playlists and indulge in some serious throwback dancing.
- Make a list of all the films you've not seen but would like to – or go through IMDb's top-ranked films and get to work!

The point is to make time for those things in your quiet moments, rather than sitting and watching other people spend their time doing the things they love.

THE JOY OF MISSING OUT

We've all experienced the dreaded calendar clash when a family event means you'll have to miss out on a friend's birthday, or the work summer bash that you've been looking forward to for months. It's easy to feel like we're the only one not in on the action, but sometimes it's about enjoying doing something with your family that you can look back on, and knowing you can catch up with work colleagues another time. Sometimes it's the things that mean we miss out which others wish they had going on themselves – no matter how uneventful they might feel to us. How many times have you been at the pub, found yourself on someone's Instagram story from their sofa, and thought, 'Wow, I wish I was inside crashing out.' When you feel like the grass is always greener, try to enjoy what you're doing in that moment and start embracing a bit of JOMO every now and again.

FOCUS ON YOU (AND YOU ONLY, LADY)

Ambition comes in all different shapes and sizes; money and textbook 'success stories' aren't the be-all and end-all. Remembering that people are driven by different incentives can help you realise that actually there is room to take your foot off the pedal, stop to smell the roses, and focus on where *you* want to be, not where *she* is.

. . . .

'Before going to university I was always made to feel as if I needed to have large aspirations. Since going through university and into work as a teacher, I've always approached it as something I'll do for as long as it feels right, which is almost frowned upon. Tutors and colleagues often assume that every good teacher's 'end goal' is to pile up as many titles, year groups or responsibilities as possible, or go into leadership – and that just isn't true for many. Having so many powerful women to look up to in 2019 is incredible and the #GirlBoss movement is very necessary and inspiring, but also sometimes makes me feel a little bit lazy. I am definitely more of a 'life'-orientated person and could never put my job fully in front of something to do with family, friends, health or wellbeing. Some days I wish I was more of a career girl, but I'm not and that's also OK!'

GEMMA, London

. . . .

The only competition you have is with yourself; the only benchmarks you should be observing are your own. Although it sounds obvious, remember that you can't change someone else's following or success, online or off. Being angry that someone else got a promotion won't bring yours on quicker. I missed out on a job at Topshop to a girl in my form at school, and I felt so envious, but then I realised that feeling that way wouldn't help me get a job there. Focusing on what other people are doing won't change the likelihood or speed of your success, so stay in your lane, girl – you got this!

Write a list of your own goals and personal ambitions (no matter how big or small) to refer to when you find yourself looking at others achieving theirs. Remember what drives you and what it is you're aiming for. It could be:

- The name of the company you've always wished to work for, be it for a one-off freelance gig or in a permanent role.
- A savings target, with a note on how much you're aiming to set aside each month.
- The number of times you intend to go for a run each week.
- That dreamy hotel you'd love to stay at.

No matter how long or short your list is, it will be a useful way of reminding yourself what it is you're driven by. Pin it up somewhere you can see it every day so you can keep it in mind.

FIND YOUR MAGIC HOUR

It's easy to assume that everyone hops out of bed at 6 a.m., grabs their NutriBullet blender for a quick protein shake, packs their pre-prepped lunch before cycling to the gym, and then hot-desks five projects until 7 p.m. But accepting that this might not be the way you live is a blessing. Having a good idea of realistic timings in your work arsenal can be the difference between a productive day and hours wasted. I've always been someone who thrives creatively in the evenings (she says, typing at 8.30 p.m. on a school night). I remember finishing my A-level history coursework at 2 a.m. the morning it was due in (Ru, my wonderful editor, I promise I won't do this to you), but that was just the time I *got shit done*. I'm not suggesting you flip your entire schedule on its head to accommodate those antisocial spurts of productivity – but if you recognise you don't get much done before midday, assign the menial tasks to your mornings. Tackle your emails, edit your photos, run to the post office, and save the later hours for the jobs that will require a little more brainpower. Of course, the same applies vice versa: if you're an early bird, get the creative juices flowing early and step away from your computer in the afternoon if you can. One person's successful working hours don't have to be yours.

CAN THE GREEN-EYED MONSTER EVER BE A WELCOME GUEST?

I never thought there would come a time when I'd be sitting down and wondering whether jealousy could truly be used as a tool for good. In the moment, it's easy to feel a twitch of jealousy after seeing someone post 'had worse Mondays' surrounded by a clear blue ocean on holiday, whilst you're sitting on the delayed 7.21 a.m. train to work. Even seeing someone collect the keys for their first house, or get a full house of A*s in their exams, can trigger jealousy. But using that feeling productively, rather than allowing it to make you feel worse, is where your power lies. On paper it sounds simple.

You could: See someone having a great time on holiday, boil up with jealousy, close Instagram and melt into a sulk for the next few hours, letting if affect your productivity, mood and interaction with others.

Or you could: See someone having a great time on holiday, boil up with jealousy, post a comment saying, 'Wish I was there! Have the best time,' close Instagram, pop on your favourite playlist and do something you like to make your day better, and nip it in the bud there and then.

Using jealousy to identify when someone else has something you strive for, rather than getting angry or upset, can help you recognise your own goals. It's OK to say, 'I'm envious of her success because she's doing what I want to do,' or, 'I'm jealous she's on holiday because I really need

71

to book a break.' Being able to admit this means we can accept that there is enough success and enjoyment for all of us, and then establish what our goals really are. Rather than getting caught up in the bitterness of someone else's achievements, congratulating them (even if from afar), acknowledging that this might be the kind of thing you'd like to aim for, and then reaching for it is a far more helpful process. Just because someone else has achieved it, doesn't mean you aren't going to. Achievements aren't limited edition! I have one of my favourite sayings on this topic pinned above my desk:

> *What's for you won't pass by you. We can't get what we want all of the time. And we can't always get it at the moment when we want it. But that doesn't mean it's not coming at all.*

When jealousy and comparison strike, I always make an effort to do something that will get me further and enrich me instead. For example, I'll read that *Stylist* article I didn't quite finish on the way home, or text a friend to check in on them. Or even better, I'll check in on myself! 'Time spent better elsewhere' has never been more applicable.

What we say *vs* what we should say

I wish I did as much travelling as she did – her life looks perfect.
I'd love to go away more this year – maybe I should plan something to look forward to.

I feel so useless. I should have bought a house by now – everyone else my age seemingly has.
I've got so much to be proud of. I wish there wasn't an expectation for people my age to tick certain boxes – I don't even necessarily want to buy a house right now!

Ugh, can you believe she got another job promotion? I wanted one!
That's great she got another promotion – I really want to aim for one too! Maybe I should plan a meeting with my manager, or set myself some steps to getting there.

I didn't deserve to get this job – they're going to realise I'm no good sooner or later.
YES! I got the job! I'm scared, but I'm so happy they went with me. It's going to be a challenge, but I know I'll learn so much.

IMPOSTER WHO?

When it comes to tackling imposter syndrome, I try to think of it as a backwards marker for how well I'm truly doing. Although I'm typing this with hindsight (and on a day when I happen to be feeling totally within my means *and* sans period hormones), sometimes I think the reason we suffer from imposter syndrome is because things are going well. Although you might not believe it, or think of yourself as deserving, you *are* in your class, at your job or hosting that event because someone (your boss or tutor, let's say) thinks you deserve to be. Your capabilities are being trusted; you haven't fooled anyone into getting to where you are. Nobody would ask you to take on something they didn't have faith you could do. Any failures or blips that happen are part of your development and the learning curve of life, and don't make you any less able or valid than before.

If you know you'll veer into imposter territory, keep a list handy – or start one (yup, this girl loves a list) – with all the little wins you feel proud of, as you experience them: a job promotion, acing a test, learning a skill, or something you saved up for. Having little pats on the back to refer to will hope-

fully make you feel like you are getting there and capable, even when it feels like you aren't. Here are some nudges in the right direction:
- Today I . . .
- Even though I was feeling low, I managed to . . .
- I was brave enough to . . .
- I made a little bit of time to . . .
- I treated myself to . . .

Whether it's sending an email where you'd normally apologise profusely and didn't, finally making time for that overdue dentist appointment (self-care in the most traditional sense) or securing a new client at work – they all deserve their own little celebration!

Takeaway pick-me-ups for kicking comparison, from The Insecure Girls' Club

- If you can't unfollow, mute anyone on social media who makes you feel unhappy, unsuccessful or uninspired.
- Start checking out your own markers for your little wins, rather than checking others' for theirs.
- Start each day, if you can, without checking your phone. Become familiar with your own company and the things you like.

- If you're scrolling as a means of procrastination, and find yourself comparing – put the phone DOWN. Instead think about how good you'll feel after you've done the task in hand.
- Remember that there are probably elements of your life that others aspire to. Perhaps you're freelance, have a great friendship group or fun relationship. Someone is probably comparing themself to you at this very moment – and the grass definitely isn't always greener.
- Remember that you and whoever you are comparing yourself to are totally different people living different lives, with different tastes and different markers of success. Their biggest goal might be writing a novel, or starring in a television show when you didn't even consider drama at GCSE! Fear not. You have brilliant qualities too – and that's what makes you interesting.

3

'I wish my body looked like that': unpicking body image

Treating ourselves the way we treat others – but only if it's nicely, of course

Here's something I hadn't thought about until recently: your body is your very own house – minus the ridiculous tenants' fees and cramped space of a one-bed city flat. It keeps you warm, safe, alive, and carries you through the difficulties, challenges, and ups and downs of life and growing up. It helps get you through break-ups with bad boyfriends, protects you from the flu you picked up wearing nothing but a beer jacket on a night out, and gets you up (albeit sometimes reluctantly) every morning for work.

But sometimes, that house has a difficult landlord. A puzzled, unreasonable homeowner that takes those things for granted. Who becomes fixated not on the house's functionality and purpose, but how it looks and how others might look at it – and suddenly that becomes far more important than what's going on inside.

Before my metaphor goes too far, I want to ask: why

and when do we start questioning everything about our body – this home – on such a superficial level? Why do all our amazing qualities quickly become boiled down to our exterior and whether it meets the expectations of not only ourselves, but the impossible ones of others too? Why do we sit online, admiring people who have access to the world's most elite personal trainers, expert dieticians, surgeons, stylists, management teams, hairstylists and make-up artists – and make it those people who we inevitably choose to consciously pit ourselves against? It's an unattainable standard that we'll never be able to reach – so why do we do it? With a new online survey conducted by the Mental Health Foundation finding that a third of adults have felt anxious because of body image concerns,[17] it's clear the pressure we're applying to ourselves, led by social media, is unsustainable and completely unjust.

> **When did you first (if ever) feel aware of how your body looked?**
>
> 'Aged twelve. A boy I'd been texting called me "the Big One". From then on, I was constantly aware of how I looked and what people thought of me.' *Grace, Sevenoaks*

For me, other than that initial comment about my ears, there certainly wasn't one standout moment when I started becoming aware of the way my body looked. It was a sour cocktail of moments that told me, from about the age of eleven (when I started secondary school), that – strangely to me, yet according to society – my body wasn't purely there for functionality. It was hearing the conversations of relatives weighing themselves on the bathroom scales that suggested self-worth could be defined by a number. Believing that whether or not a pair of jeans fitted could be the measure of my happiness with the way I looked (and how, from such a skewed viewpoint, it felt easier to change my whole body than to pop back to the high street to replace the damn denim). Being told, when I started developing boobs and soft curves where I had been 'straight up and down', that it was probably 'puppy fat' which I'd 'just lose anyway' – as if it was a bad thing to have in the first place.

. . . .

'I remember when a relative said, "Ah, she's lost all the puppy fat" in my early teens. We've grown up with people thinking it's OK to make flippant comments and it's really a reflection of the diet-obsessed culture we live in. I used to be obsessed with reading celebrity weights in *Heat* and comparing my measurements to models'. Now I realise how damaging that was. Remember that it's an age-old system with outdated body measurements that's the issue, not you.'

KRISTABEL, London

. . . .

From my pre-teens to my mid-twenties, rather than disappearing like immature boyfriends and a now wavering love for boy bands and McFly, those feelings of body uncertainty simply evolved. I covered my walls with magazine cut-outs as I turned sixteen, and became infatuated with pictures of Alexa Chung at Glastonbury that would have me yearning for supermodel-length pin-up legs (even though my genetic make-up, with both parents under 5'9", would never allow for that). I should have left my Cindy Crawford/Twiggy dreams in my fluffy pink Groovy Chick diary where they belonged, and focused on the more important things – like how to ever access a Busted meet-and-greet.

However, I recognise that I'm still in an enormously privileged position when it comes to my body. I am an able-bodied, white, slim woman who is able to go into Topshop and pick out something in her size with minimal fuss. I am able to recognise models in shop windows who look similar to me, and my shape is very rarely (if ever) scrutinised on the front of trashy women's magazines. I don't have to worry that if a mannequin is produced in my size in a popular sports shop, it will be met with derision. Being in a body that isn't marginalised by the media is a sad privilege; the heartbreaking fact that certain body shapes are more 'accepted' by the media is something that shouldn't be the reality.

But know that your body – however small, big, tall, short or physically able – truly does not define you. The way you look is not what is most important. As body positive advocate Megan Jayne Crabbe says, 'Nobody loves you more than your body. Every cell is here for you' – and isn't that the truth. Your body really is your biggest fan.

OUR BODIES, ONLINE

Just think – if you were never to post another pic-
ture of yourself on holiday in a bikini on Instagram
ever again, would you still fret as much before going
away?

The same goes for if you woke up and genuinely didn't care about the way your body looked – what would you do differently? If it was a nice day, would you wear those shorts you've been 'reserving for when you lose weight'? Would you ask that total catch (who says 'catch' anymore?) on a date that you've been putting off? Or would you feel confident enough to finally get up in your favourite pub and sing karaoke, knowing that the thing that's always stopped you never needed to in the first place?

Looking through old pictures recently has made me so aware of how attuned to our physical quirks the internet can make us. Although viral posts like the #10yearchallenge can provide positive hindsight and a solid dose of 'Why didn't I appreciate how good I looked?' perspective, the Be Real Campaign (a national movement made up of individuals, schools, businesses and charities that is determined to change attitudes to body image) recently discovered that more than two-thirds of young people feel pressure to look their best online, with the same number editing photos of themselves before posting).[18] Every day we are presented with feeds of impossible ideals, with articles debating those ideals and the conversation around body confidence, image and dieting ever present.

. . . .

'As I grew older I was introduced to social media (Facebook, Instagram, etc.) which vastly narrowed my image of beauty. "I must be three times smaller in size to even potentially be considered pretty! My face must be flawless without make-up! I must have no fat rolls or cellulite! I must be a goddess to be accepted!" The worst words I put upon myself were "I must". I didn't have to be any of those things to be me and be beautiful.'

BEX, Huddersfield

. . . .

There are things about my body that I've only started to notice in the last few years – the dimples on my elbows that I always thought should be on my cheeks, and my dad's athletic legs (which I've grown to love and remind me of him). These are things I've only been made aware of due to strangers online projecting their own negative perceptions and insecurities onto me. Emily, a member of The Insecure Girls' Club from the Philippines, says, 'It's crazy, because being athletic, I used to love how my body was capable of so many physical activities. But when I started to look at myself through the eyes of a boy I wanted to please, I saw all the flaws that weren't there before.' We're so used to taking a photograph for Instagram, and then zooming in to inspect every facet of our body to check it's up to an invisible standard. A bar subliminally set to no real height, and one we will probably never allow ourselves to reach.

. . . .

'I'm quite short with pale, freckled skin and ginger hair. I used to feel quite self-conscious about that but it's been great seeing a greater variety of bodies online and on TV in the last few years.'

JASMINE, London

. . . .

On holiday last year, I remember becoming aware that the photos I was taking of myself in a bikini were for nothing more than an Instagram post. I'd had a brilliant day lounging on the beach, headphones in and sand between my toes – laughing into my Fanta Limón and guzzling my bodyweight in aioli. But the moment it came down to was this: the posed bikini photograph that never made the cut because it wasn't how I thought it should look. It wasn't a moment I was keen on documenting, but I'd felt obliged to share it to tick a 'social media holiday box'. Then, amidst the endless scrolling, comparison and tidal wave of bikini pictures, before-and-afters and heavily Photoshopped glamazons, something hit me: I don't want to look at old photographs and have the first thing I notice be my ever-softening jawline.

I don't want my bone structure to be the value I place on a memory that was worth so much more than that. I don't take a photograph to capture how my body looks, but to document something far more significant – a memory, time spent with someone special, or a holiday postcard moment to look back on. Yet with the job of being an 'online content creator', the pressure to document every moment increases. Is it good enough to just share silly holiday snaps? Do I have to match this standard because it's 'expected' of me? Do I need to constantly subscribe to the 'photos or it didn't happen' perspective? The pressure to abide by the unwritten rules can feel enormous, even if you know all too well that to be happy and content in your body does not mean you have to share it in swimwear online.

A CLOTHING SIZE DOESN'T COME WITH A CONFIDENCE TAG

Body image is such a delicate subject, because nobody can write about it from any perspective other than their own. Nobody knows the way you feel about your body like you do; nobody can question that relationship – and no matter who you are, everyone is entitled to feel insecure in their body and experience their own personal hang-ups.

. . . .

'Sometimes it does feel a bit taboo to say that you don't feel good in your own body because we are bombarded with a "body confidence" wave. And as great as this is, I do feel ashamed to say that no, I don't always love my body.'

LESLIE, France

. . . .

I once received an Instagram message saying: 'If you have bikini worries yet you are a size 6–10 you're not that relatable, hun.' Firstly, I believe *anyone* can feel self-conscious about their body, no matter what their size (which isn't saying you *should*, because if you don't that's brill)! I have friends and family of all sizes who have felt equally insecure at various points in their lives, whatever the number inside the T-shirt they're wearing might be – because unfortunately, a clothing size doesn't come with a confidence tag. As fashion stylist Grace Woodward said, 'When we stopped getting clothes via makers and started buying standardised sizing, we started to diminish the uniqueness of our bodies. We had to fit the clothes, not the other way round.'[19]

There is nothing stickier than an 'Oh, but other people have it harder' mindset: everybody's insecurities are both relative and valid, with the way we view our body being just one of them. We need to stop assuming that people are or should be ashamed of their body, and that if someone looks a certain way they should be confident.

> **Do you feel the bodies you see on TV represent you?**
>
> 'I am a fat wheelchair user – there are so few wheelchair users on TV, and when there are they tend to be in the Paralympics. It feels like people only want to see "inspirational" disabled people.' *Anna, Cambridge*

In a world that champions slim, toned women on magazine covers, advertising and catwalk shows, it's easy to assume that nobody who, in our eyes, has a more 'desirable' figure could ever feel insecure. I've looked at people in the past, people with a different frame from me, and questioned *how on earth* they could ever be unhappy with their body. The same way I've looked at people with thousands of followers online and wondered how anybody like that could ever be lonely, or feel discontent. But, honestly? You never know what's going on behind closed doors; the struggles people are experiencing, the conversations they've had or the turbulence they've felt. Conversely, you might sometimes think you've no right to feel insecure, but trust me, you are well within your rights – it's just a case of being tactful about how you project those insecurities, and ensuring that when the topic of body image comes up, you're not making someone else feel insecure about themselves too. Which leads me nicely on to . . .

HOW WE TALK TO OURSELVES
(AND OTHERS) MATTERS

One of the most positive things you can do for your body is to look at the way you talk about it: be it to yourself pre-shower, in front of your bedroom mirror as you have a night-before outfit-panic, online, or – arguably most importantly – to anyone else. My favourite episode of Fearne Cotton's *Happy Place* podcast was her conversation with Davina McCall. When discussing the big life lessons she's learnt, Davina openly says hers is 'to love yourself – a much harder lesson than I ever thought it would be. I always had this idea in my twenties that loving yourself was this kind of terrible, arrogant thing to do, and "Ugh, how cocky!" To say that you love yourself!' She then goes on to share honestly how, at a low point, her sponsor gave her a mirror and asked her to say 'I like you' out loud to it every day. It took weeks of work for her to get there, showing it's truly all about practice. She says, 'She helped me get to the point where I thought, "I'm worthy of love," and that's the thing, isn't it – to love yourself or to be loved, you have to feel worthy of love.'[20]

Although sharing is caring, and sharing our stories and insecurities is fundamental to making each other feel less alone, when it comes to body image, being careful with our language is paramount to ensuring the conversation never makes anyone else feel 'less than'.

Has someone else criticising themselves ever
made you worry about yourself?

Yes: 98% | No: 1% | Don't know: 1%

Have you ever been in a situation where you thought, 'God, if they're thinking that about themselves, then what must they think about me?!' I remember being on a trip with someone who commented endlessly on the size of her thighs. To me they were as good as thighs got – not only did they help carry her from A to B (which, let's be honest, is their primary function), but they were also toned, lengthy, and could rival some of those on the magazine cut-outs I'd had on my wall growing up. To say I was envious would be completely accurate. However, she hated them. She commented endlessly on the size of them, how 'big' they seemed to her, how much she disliked the way they looked – which of course she was entitled to feel, except it started making me question my own legs. Having thighs comfortably double the size of hers, I began analysing my own, and developed a self-consciousness that pretty much directly rubbed off hers. To me this wasn't about body size, but rather the words she chose to speak to herself and how that insecurity projected itself onto me. Of course, these throwaway comments are never made with malice. I know I've spoken about my body negatively in the past – picking out 'flaws' with friends and having a good moan in the midst of a confidence wobble. But it's the thought I might have made someone else feel 'less than' that makes my stomach sink. It's something we all should all be able to talk about, but being careful and considerate with our language should always be primary.

BODIES AND 'THE BIG DAY'

Losing weight and 'making changes to ourselves' are so intrinsically connected with 'big occasions'. Whether that's the opening of an exhibition you've curated, your first gig as a musician, your graduation, or presenting a game-changing pitch to a new client, unsolicited pressure to 'improve' ourselves can creep up, or be drip-fed to us without us even realising. It's almost normalised – and I hadn't really thought about it until I started planning my own 'big day'. When I got engaged, one of the first questions that started popping up when trying on bridal dresses was whether I intended to lose weight for the wedding.

'So, are you planning on dieting before the big day?' I'd be asked by a bridal shop assistant – as casually as asking whether I caught last night's *X Factor* on TV. 'Oh, that's normal, right?' I initially thought, before feeling disappointed that the body I'd been comfortable in up until now was perhaps not what it 'should' be ahead of one of the most important days of my life. Should I have started a strict exercise regime before now? Should I have been food prepping my way into my wedding dress?

It's only looking back at those flippant remarks now that I realise the gravity and weight they held. What's wrong with my body as it is? Why should I need to change it for a party?

Wedding or otherwise, I've never wanted to get toned or exercise to look better, but rather to feel comfortable enough for my body not to be the focal point of my thoughts. If I choose to exercise, it's because I want to become healthier, stronger or fitter, as opposed to losing a chunk of it (which doesn't always equate to being healthier) – so I can get on with life, and not make my body the epicentre. And isn't that what body confidence is? Feeling confident enough in yourself that any doubts you have around your body don't affect your overall performance.

After applying a lot of pressure to myself to change how I looked because I thought I had to, something clicked inside. I didn't need to drop a dress size, 'get lean' in how- ever many days, or do a full Trinny-and-Susannah-style makeover, because I was lucky enough to be getting mar- ried. It was like a light had gone on and I realised my body was absolutely fine as it was. Yes, I still had moments of insecurity – when I noticed the dimples, ripples and lines in my skin that sometimes I didn't always love – but for who I am, nothing needed to change.

GETTING COSY WITH YOURSELF

But of course, confidence isn't something we can just switch on and off. No matter what body we're in, sometimes knowing we should love ourselves wholly and unconditionally is a pressure in itself. It can take a lifetime to nurture, and some days it'll come more effortlessly than others. It's easier said than done and, like performing the full dance routine to 'Single Ladies', it requires a fair bit of rehearsal.

Sometimes I think the kindest way to start is to treat yourself as if you were little again. As if you were a parent looking after a small you. Remember those pictures from when you were a toddler? The ones you'd use for a #TBT on Instagram? The 'Oh my God, look how *cute* I was!' ones? Look after that person – because really, they're still the same. Feed yourself proper meals, recognise when you've had too much screen time (even if these days it's probably more scrolling and less *SMTV Live*), and take yourself out for fresh air and walks when you start to get stir-crazy indoors. There's a lot to be said for the way we treat children, and sometimes that care, nurture and kindness is all we need to give ourselves too.

I saw a brilliant mantra on Instagram recently from Anuschka Rees, author of *Beyond Beautiful*, a book that encourages us to shift the way we think about our body to a more neutral sense, and shows that what's most important isn't anything to do with being attractive. She said, 'My appearance is going to shape-shift a million times throughout my life. Sometimes I'll find myself more attractive, sometimes less so. And that's OK.'[21]

And that's exactly it. Being OK with having mixed feelings, some good days, some less so, and still being able to get up and get on with the day. Being able to take a compliment, enjoy it (because hey, we're only human) when someone says you look nice – but not being totally reliant on those compliments to keep you thriving. Being able to look back at old photos and remember who you were with, what you were doing and how you felt in that moment is so much more important that remembering what size dress you had on. Being neither here nor there about the way our body looks, putting emotion to one side, and switching over negative thoughts to compassionate, cosy ones which remind us that our body is just that – a body.

Nadia Craddock
body image researcher

So, how can we start developing the steps to a healthier relationship with our body, whilst battling insecurity? I spoke to the inspiring and incredibly wise Nadia Craddock – a PhD candidate at the Centre for Appearance Research (CAR) and host of *Appearance Matters* and *The Body Protest* podcasts, to discuss how we can improve the way we view our body – and how society impacts our thinking, often without us realising . . .

Nadia, you've been involved in a number of incredible projects connected to improving body image – how did you become interested in body image research?
To be honest, I kind of (very fortunately) fell into it and never looked back. I didn't know body image research was a thing five years ago. I was at Harvard doing a Master's in human development and psychology and I wasn't exactly sure what the next move was. I definitely didn't see myself working in academia *at all*. But towards the end of spring semester, I went to a talk by my now PhD supervisor, about her work on an evidence-based body image curriculum that was being

delivered in 100+ countries around the world, in partnership with the World Association of Girl Guides and Girl Scouts and the Dove Self-Esteem Project, and I was hooked. After I graduated, I moved back to the UK and I worked on that project for a year before transitioning to my PhD.

Your work goes into the depths of developing a body-positive attitude and helping people have a healthier relationship with their body; from big brands to individuals, how do you define positive body image?

I'm glad you asked this! Positive body image (as we talk about it in research, at least) is defined as feelings of care, respect, appreciation and acceptance towards your body, regardless of how it matches up to societal beauty standards, as well as a sense of connectedness to your body. In this way, positive body image is much more than simply thinking you look good. I mean, don't get me wrong – thinking you look good is great, but it's what I would probably refer to as 'body confidence' and/or 'body satisfaction' in a research context.

I think it's also worth saying that having a positive body image doesn't mean that you will never have any negative body image thoughts or a bad body image day. Given the society we live in and all the appearance pressures out there, that might be a little unrealistic. Having a positive body image means that you are in a better place to not let negative thoughts affect you.

Another thing that is important to mention is that positive body image is distinct from the body positivity movement. The body positivity movement is a social, political collective effort to amplify and give space to bodies that are marginalised and oppressed in society, to include fat bodies, black and brown bodies, trans bodies, disabled bodies, etc. People are fighting for basic respect, and I think it's important for people with more body privilege to be cognisant of that.

You host a wonderful, research-based, education-fuelled podcast and cover everything from diet culture and eating disorders to the language we use and social media. What is the biggest lesson you've learnt since talking about all these facets that make up body image?
Thanks for the kind words about the podcast; I'm so proud of it. I think it's so important for people in academia to share knowledge and learnings, which is what we are trying to do with the pod. A couple of recent standout episodes for me were with Dr Jerel Calzo and Dr Allegra Gordon, talking about sexual identity and gender identity respectively on body image and disordered eating. Both Jerel and Allegra talk about how the experience of discrimination and stigma impact how people relate to their bodies. This has been one of my biggest learnings – body image concerns are not just the product of looking at skinny models. Racism, fatphobia, homophobia, transphobia, ableism, etc. all can play a role.

What would be your one piece of advice to someone currently struggling with their own body image insecurities?
I think one of the most important things to remember is that your body is not the problem and you are so, SO much more than your body. Focus on your values, qualities and interests beyond your body and immerse yourselves in those.

LET'S RECAP!

....

And breathe! After delving deep into reels of Instagram bikini photos and asking when we started seeing our bodies as anything more than the functioning miracles they are, it's clear that body image is a topic with endless questions, and a tapestry of threads that might never fully be unpicked. We've explored how unattainable standards on and offline, and the expectations we set ourselves (plus shaking them off with a hair-flip of reality) tie in with the impact of social media and how body confidence certainly isn't a one-size-fits-all.

STOP RIGHT NOW, THANK YOU VERY MUCH

So, where do we go from here when it comes to picking each other up, recognising that we're enough as we are, and appreciating ourselves as much as we appreciate Armie Hammer and Timothée Chalamet in *Call Me By Your Name*? Ahem . . .

CHANGE YOUR PERSPECTIVE

Although the conversation around body image online can feel noisy and overwhelming (and sometimes like it's drawing even more attention to the way we look, rather than just letting us be), there are spaces popping up that flip the perspective on its head, leaving us with the feeling that, actually, we're enough as we are. We're in charge of who we follow on Instagram (and whether we want to use social media at all): swapping in someone more inspiring who makes us feel better is an easy thing to achieve.

In 2018, Jameela Jamil created 'I Weigh' (@i_weigh), an inclusive platform that celebrates the weight of women's values and achievements, after an image showing each Kardashian member's body weight went viral. A whole new movement began, showcasing the real metrics we should be focusing on: our personality qualities (creative, funny, brave), hobbies (painting, tennis, running), life experiences (mother, graduate, survivor), relationships we value (loving girlfriend, sister, cousin), challenges we've been through and accomplishments we've achieved; and emphasising that it's these things we should be shouting about – not the little number that looks up at us from a set of scales.

Although it often can be, the internet doesn't have to be a trigger for negative self-thoughts. There are so many incredible body positive advocates online who are changing the way we use social media for the greater good.

There are brilliant people doing the work online to make us all feel more body confident. I've included a list of my favourite accounts in The Insecure Girl's Library on page 233, but for further scrolling may I recommend:

- @calliethorpe
- @bodyposipanda
- @stylemesunday
- @torie_snelvis
- @munroebergdorf
- @nerdabouttown
- @bryonygordon
- @celestebarber
- @itstrinanicole
- @jess_megan_

And if in doubt, here are a few things your bodyweight doesn't factor in:

- Happiness
- The hard times
- The side-splittingly wonderful times
- The last song you learnt all the lyrics to
- Your favourite party trick
- The Little Mix dance you know all the moves to
- Your expression when you're hysterically happy from laughing

- The satisfaction of cooking your favourite dinner at home
- The achievement of trying something new
- The feeling you get after the short walk home instead of taking a taxi
- How brilliant you are, as you are

Megan Jayne Crabbe

body positive advocate, author and wonder woman behind the @bodyposipanda blog

If you haven't discovered Megan on Instagram yet, where have you been? Since starting @bodyposipanda, Megan has been a true influence for change – sharing and discussing body positivity, intuitive eating and confidence online as well as writing the bestselling book *Body Positive Power* . . .

Megan, your page has been one of my absolute favourites to follow on Instagram for a long time, and I know that I (as well as thousands of others) always come away feeling better than when I arrived – which is what it's all about. What inspired you to start sharing your story so openly online?

The simple answer to this is that I found something that changed my life and I needed to share it with as many people as possible. I'd spent the majority of my life fighting against my body, either obsessively dieting or battling eating disorders. Then at the age of twenty-one I stumbled across the body positive movement online – it was a small community of people with bodies of all shapes and sizes talking about accepting themselves, no longer dieting, and refusing to believe that how they looked was all they had to offer the world. I never knew before that point that accepting myself was even an option. My Instagram page really started as a personal journal, just me documenting my own healing and connecting with a community of people doing the same. The more people who found me and told me that they'd felt the same things, the more I realised how important it was for me to keep spreading the message as far as I possibly could. It's a profoundly beautiful thing to be able to turn your own painful experiences into something healing for other people, and I feel incredibly grateful to be able to have done that.

How has sharing your journey and story changed the way you view yourself and your body?
When I started posting pictures of my own body, I was really determined to romanticise all the physical parts of myself that I'd spent so long hating. I used exposure to photos of myself to make peace with the softness of my stomach, to celebrate the cellulite on my thighs, to embrace every bit of jiggle in videos of myself dancing. I needed to aim for love, because the hate was always so powerful it felt like I needed as much strength in the opposite direction to make the shift. These days it's less about being visually in love with myself, and more about knowing that I've always been so much more than any body part. I've travelled through body hatred and body love to land on body neutrality most days, and I'm definitely happiest here.

I think for a lot of people, you changed the way they used social media when it came to comparison and body image – which is amazing and so powerful. What's been the biggest lesson you've learnt since starting @bodyposipanda?

That change happens through the culmination of millions of tiny actions. One of my favourite people to follow is Rachel Cargle (@rachel.cargle), and she writes beautifully about the effect of ripples, and how it isn't one giant action that creates a wave of change, it's all of us creating ripples in our communities that then grow bigger and less ignorable over time. Social media feels like that to me.

We all have days when we're not feeling great about ourselves, and you talk about this so much, which is reassuring. What are your top three tips for tackling a down day?

Allow yourself to feel whatever you're feeling. My relationship with my own mental health changed so much when I shifted from, 'Why do I have to feel this way?' to, 'I feel this way and that's OK.' Darker days are much easier to weather without the added guilt and shame of blaming yourself for the darkness. Do things that have absolutely nothing to do with how your body looks – create, see friends, find the thing that brings you a tiny bit of joy, and do it even if you're not good at it or it's not necessarily productive. Be gentle with yourself, as gentle as you possibly can be.

What would be the one thing you would say to someone currently struggling with their body, or feeling insecure?

You deserve better. How you're feeling about your body right now isn't something that you've ever deserved to feel. It isn't because you haven't worked hard enough, it has nothing to do with willpower, and it isn't just the way things are. You feel this way about your body because we live in a culture that conditions us to see our bodies as flawed and imperfect, because our insecurities can easily be turned into profit for the biggest industries in the world ready to sell us the solution to imperfection. You didn't ask for any of this, and neither did your body – it's just trying to carry you through life as best it can. And even if you can't make peace with your body right now, please know that you deserve better than a life spent at war with yourself, because we all do.

Finally, as a woman with lots of wise words and brilliant mantras, do you have any words to live by that members of The Insecure Girls' Club can add to their repertoire?
Allow yourself to be human. Apologise for your existence less. Feel your feelings. Make mistakes. Know that you're not supposed to have any of it figured out. In every moment of doubt, fear, shame, joy, anger, anticipation, light and shade, you are so beautifully human. Hold on to that.

LET'S TALK ACCEPTANCE

For most of us, it's simply not natural to love our body constantly. Much like life – and our relationship with the priest from *Fleabag* – it will always have its ups and downs. And perhaps it's not about loving it constantly, but accepting it for what it is instead – warts and all. There might be bits we don't like as much as others, days when we don't feel as ready to pose as others, but accepting that is absolutely fine. Learn to talk to yourself with kindness and compassion on the days when things aren't so great, and focus on the things that you do feel good about. For example:

- I got on top of my work today.
- I did really well in that meeting this week.
- I pulled myself out of bed when I could have easily stayed there all day.
- I cooked myself a meal from scratch.
- I finally finished the last chapter of the book I've been reading all month.

Don't let one negative thought be the template for your whole day: a bad morning doesn't have to mean a bad week.

CHANGE THE CONVERSATION

If your friends and family talk about their bodies a lot, which makes you think about yours more than you would like, talk to them and ask if they can stop. Perhaps you could all agree not to weigh yourself for a month (and then carry on afterwards)? Every time they start to criticise their bodies, encourage them to say something kind instead. Maybe set up a pound jar in case you trip up, and use it towards drinks at the end of the month! Be mindful of how you compliment each other too.

Here are some of my favourite non-appearance-related compliments for inspiration:
- You are so inspiring.
- You make me feel like I can take on anything.
- I love spending time with you.
- I feel so lucky to know you.
- You're so thoughtful.
- You make me smile.
- You're a total ray of sunshine.
- You're so brilliant at your job.
- You mean a lot to me.
- You make me laugh so much.
- You make me feel loved and accepted for who I am.

- You really are the life and soul of the party.
- You are such a brilliant pal.
- You are so funny.
- You're one of the coolest people I know.
- You light up a room.
- I'd trust you to look after my dog (we all know how much of a compliment that is!).

Also, let's all admit we sometimes have a bitchy leak and try to stop doing that too. Every time you think something negative about somebody, remind yourself in a kind way that if you keep looking at other people like that, you'll keep looking at yourself like that too. These are habits we have to learn to break, but by pulling ourselves (and others) up gently, we can re-learn the best way to talk to others and ourselves.

You are not a bag of flour in a cake recipe; you don't need to be measured on a set of scales.

PERFECT AS YOU ARE RIGHT NOW, PAL

Like a great sequinned mini dress or the fancy-as Chloé bag you saved up hard for, your body shouldn't be saved for 'best'. Make the most of it now. Stop waiting to try something new, take a dance class, or wear the outfit that's been gathering dust in your wardrobe until you've lost weight – we don't need to wait to start enjoying life, because it's ready to be enjoyed just as we are. Our bodies are not a work in progress. We are complete and ready to go right now, and by waiting for things to change we could be waiting a long time. Our expectations will continually shift and change, and one day I can promise you'll look back and wonder why you didn't enjoy those moments when they were there. So, get up and dust yourself off, because you are perfect as you are right now.

WHEN IN DOUBT, BE A REBEL

That doesn't mean sticking chewing gum under the table in McDonald's – it means being rebellious by feeling good about your body. In a world that ultimately benefits from us worrying about the way we look – companies cash in from our desire to 'improve' our body – loving yourself exactly as you are is the most powerful middle finger you can show to those standards (in addition to saving your money, which they would've preferred you to spend on anti-cellulite cream, fillers or expensive waxes). Self-love isn't something to be monetised – it's so much more than a fancy facial or manicure. Knowing you don't have to change a single thing about yourself is the biggest act of self-love.

Takeaway pick-me-ups for ultimate outside-in feel good, from The Insecure Girls' Club

- Take care of yourself. Look out for yourself the way you would your very best friend. If your body is asking for an early night, give it one. Run yourself a bath, light a candle and order a pizza. You are the best person to supply self-love; make yourself a priority and talk to yourself as you would the people you think the world of.
- Praise yourself before waiting for others' approval. If you feel great, you are great. Don't wait for someone else to confirm it before you can enjoy the feeling.
- Pay attention to the way you talk to your body. Check that the language you use to yourself is the kind of language you'd use to talk to anyone else. Remember, best to be kind, and neutral as the default.
- Realise it's OK to have mixed feelings. We won't always love the way we look – and that's OK. It doesn't make us better or worse people. Having mixed feelings about your body doesn't have to be self-defining – some days you'll like things, some days you won't. That's normal and we all feel the same way.
- Take the bar away. Realise you don't have to set a bar for yourself to be happy. You are not a work in progress.
- Accept that it's normal to enjoy receiving compliments, but don't become reliant on them to fuel your self-esteem. If a selfie doesn't rack up thirty comments, or if

the first thing your pal says to you isn't 'You look nice', that's not the be-all and end-all. Your value is more than what someone else thinks of you.

What is the one thing you like most about your body?

'That it works! Every day I remind myself that my hands let me make art, my brain can focus on the tasks ahead and my legs get me from one area to another. It's amazing.'

Anon

4

'But do you think I offended her?':
pressing mute on your constant
inner worrier

Challenging the negative monologue after
any new or difficult social interaction

I'd been at a gorgeous candle-lit dinner. Feasting amongst flowers that probably cost the same as a small flat, with a menu only a *MasterChef* contestant could conjure up, and surrounded by women far more glamorous than me, who for once I hadn't felt totally intimidated by. I was chatting away, pulling out my favourite dad jokes, and feeling quietly confident that I'd done a 'good job' at being social.

But within hours of arriving home, I was mentally back at the table replaying everything. My internal cinema had set up a showing of *Everything You Did Wrong Tonight* and I was in the starring role. Had I been too outspoken? Did people think I just love the sound of my own voice? God, I must have laughed so much at my own jokes. They must think I'm so annoying and will never invite me to anything again! Before I knew it, I assumed I'd been struck off the guest list for any future events, believed everyone was snidely laughing at anything I said, and had completely lost perspective on how the evening had actually gone.

And it's not just after posh dinners that these things happen. Insecurity often waits until we're alone with our thoughts, when we start picking at ourselves like flecks of chipped nail varnish. More often than not, it comes after a quick interaction with someone new, or conversations with friends. It happens at work or at school. It's the narrative we subliminally create to make problems that aren't there in the first place. Online it's even worse – things can get so swiftly taken out of context, with unanswered 'read' messages leaving us wondering what we've done wrong.

The negative back-chat we have with ourselves isn't affected by our age, life experience or the number of friends we have. It's ready to pluck the most insignificant comments and turn them into something far more impactful, leading to bouts of anxiety that we certainly could all do without.

THE SERIAL SECOND-GUESSER

For a long time, I'd sit and worry about situations I'd left feeling perfectly fine, breaking them down until a murky taste of uncertainty was the only thing that was left. It didn't matter whether it was because my reaction to a friend's new haircut was too slow (a 0.1-second delay before saying, 'It looks great!' was enough to launch a catastrophic meltdown in my mind) or whether I'd been 'too full-on' whilst meeting new people: the fear of what others thought – after first impressions, or time spent together – would be agonising.

Typing it now, it feels narcissistic to assume people would leave my company and immediately start talking about me, (which is perhaps another insecurity in itself, ARGH INSECURITY INCEPTION) – but as humans we're conditioned to seek approval – we water ourselves down for fear of the opinions that come afterwards. In the September 2018 issue of *Vogue*, even Beyoncé spoke about her desire to be liked(!) EVEN BEYONCÉ. She said, 'I look at the woman I was in my twenties and I see a young lady growing into confidence but intent on pleasing everyone around her.'[22] Which shows that no matter how many headliner slots we've accumulated, we've all been there.

. . . .

'I'm insecure when I make a first impression. I immediately assume that I've come off less intelligent than I am, said the wrong thing, insulted someone, or that they just downright would never want to be my friend. Why would they want to be my friend? I only pulled this cool outfit together because I saw a girl on Instagram wearing it. I'm not actually cool – it's a facade! I'M SORRY!'

MEGAN, Norwich

. . . .

113

This second-guessing is almost like an act of self-protection – 'If I think it before they do, then at least I'm prepared for the worst. GOTCHA!'

If there's one thing that hasn't changed from primary school to adulthood, it's that meeting people for the first time is scary. Seemingly, all of the things we feel most vulnerable about are on display, and it's easy to feel like they're on the table for judgement. If we're able to pick them apart first, perhaps it won't feel so bad when the other person *inevitably* sees all of those things, right? But unlike the happy-go-lucky five-year-olds in the playground meeting friends for the first time, we worry about it afterwards. They might be nervous about their first day at school, but they'd rarely panic about what Sophie thought of their new Barbie. Do you remember stepping away from meeting your primary school best friend (probably whilst picking your nose) and worrying what they thought? Of course you didn't! As a grown-up it's normal to worry about what others think (I like to believe it shows you care), but given that we're powerless to change anyone's opinion of us, it's a wasted worry.

One thing I've learnt is that worrying has never changed the outcome of a situation that has already happened. You've already put your best foot forward (and even if you haven't, there's time to apologise and move on). You can analyse your behaviour until the cows come home, but whether or not somebody likes you will never be your decision.

THE WHATSAPP WORRIER

Ever since 'read' receipts on social media were invented, being an expert over-analyser has become exceptionally easy. From the days of MSN Messenger and friendly 'nudges', feeling like you're being given the cyber cold shoulder is something we've all experienced in some way or another.

> **Have you ever stayed up late/missed a bus/been distracted by waiting to see if a message you sent has been 'read'?**
>
> Yes: 60% | No: 37% | Don't know: 3%

Take, for example, seeing that someone didn't wish you a happy birthday on Facebook and then wondering what you did wrong all those months ago. When a friend leaves you with the dreaded two blue ticks on WhatsApp after several offers to hang out, we naturally think, 'Am I *that* annoying?' before opening up endless mental manuscripts of past conversations to pinpoint what put them off. The insecure girl can always find something she did wrong and construct a problem with which to mentally torture herself.

In these moments, we forget that people are busy, have other things they're desperately juggling, or (as in my case) are just really rubbish on WhatsApp (honestly, it's a skill

I'm working on). I've done it, I have pals that have done it – and even though we can see it from both sides with a bit of perspective, when the boot is on the other foot it simply feels rude. If your closest friends never comment on your photos online but they're still checking in with you elsewhere, is that the point at which we have to have a bit of a word with ourselves and start weighing up what's truly important?

When I was growing up, I'd usually reply to texts with 'Cool!' when a social plan was organised. I didn't use bucket-fuls of expressive emojis or kisses, and often this would be interpreted as me being standoffish, uninterested and rude, with friends checking to see if they'd done anything wrong, or asking what was up. Now I have friends who sign off conversations with – wait for it – a full stop. How *curt*! They must *hate* me! But a keyboard is the breeding ground of misunderstandings, and misreading the tone of a message can be the first trap for the insecure girl. Choosing to take things at face value is the key to letting go of that worry – and realising that a little dot at the end of a sentence is usually little more than the proper use of punctuation.

Similarly, most of the time an unread message means nothing more than a struggle to keep up – it's so rarely armed with a hidden message or anything deeper. In an age where most of us have Facebook, Messenger, Twitter, Instagram, WhatsApp and iMessage on our phone, not staying on top of everything is down to busyness and forgetfulness. Social media can be incredibly overwhelming. Statistics from the Department for Culture, Media and

Sport identified that 70 per cent of adults have used social media in the last year, with 68.8 per cent using it at least once a day (and half of those using it several times a day).[23] We're constantly told not to be on our phones, to cut down on screen time and just switch off – but when our relationships are sprinkled across multiple apps, it's more realistic to learn to find the balance between being active online and maintaining our sanity.

'I CAN'T WORK OUT IF THIS IS THE RIGHT THING TO SAY' – TRUSTING OUR OWN OPINIONS

With our own negative back-chat shrouding us in self-doubt left, right and centre, having confidence in our own judgement can feel like climbing a mountain. But to channel RuPaul: if you don't have faith in yourself, how can you expect others to have faith in you? When I lived at home I was so reliant on asking my mum for a second opinion on everything, but since moving out I've had to rely on and trust my judgement more and more – and actually, it's not always completely wrong.

Online culture demands that we have the answers to everything, and a solid, informed opinion on anything we choose to discuss, making us feel silly or ill-equipped if we don't. With so many big, loud and confident voices surrounding us, it's easy to lose track of our own opinions – and when others are so sure of themselves, we can start doubting our own views if we don't have that kind of confidence; whether that's a work colleague, a journalist on Twitter, or a friend who appears to be more clued up than you.

. . . .

'I have so many conversations with female friends about the insecurities we feel in the workplace. I'm a business consultant and the need to always be "on" for my clients means there is a *lot* of pressure for someone who doubts themself a good 70 per cent of the time. Being surrounded by super-smart, confident people seems to make me doubt myself more. I'm great at my job, but I always relied on reassurance from others that I'm doing a good job to counter the voices in my head telling me that I'm not. After a lot of reflection and an attempt to focus more on my work-life balance I have made those voices quieter, need less reassurance from others and feel way more confident in myself. If you flick through my work notebook, you'll find paragraphs of my thoughts littered throughout. For me it's the best way to get the insecurities out of my head and onto the page so I can focus on what I need to do next.'

LYDIA, London

. . . .

The danger here is that we start to question ourselves: Do I know enough about this topic to talk about it? Can I hold my own enough if I start a conversation? If my boss is saying that, then she must be right and I must be wrong! We avoid the possibility of being judged for not knowing, so we stay quiet instead.

However, we cannot assume we're wrong just because of our experience, our position or our confidence. Jade, a member of The Insecure Girls' Club from Dorset, says, 'I thought if I wanted to be successful, I needed to make no mistakes and be on top form 100 per cent of the time whilst being like other people I aspired to be like.' Learning to trust your gut and admit that every mistake is part of the learning process is a valuable tool – and it means that even if you don't get it right first time, there's a positive lesson to be taken away.

ON BEING LIKED . . .

Who doesn't want to be liked by everyone they meet? It's a deep-rooted human trait to crave acceptance and approval: we evolved to survive in groups. So, when we haven't got a support network, the feeling of being disliked can be completely crushing, leading us to agonise over everything we aren't instead of focusing on everything we are. Sometimes the fear of being left out because we're blazing our own trail or doing things differently can be a worry too, and I truly don't think I know anyone that hasn't fretted about someone else's opinion of them at one point or another. I know that being the 'emo' kid in secondary school did me no favours in terms of popularity (*weird*, because I thought everyone loved listening to Bring Me the Horizon over lunch). But to me, being accepted by the people that cared was a higher priority than trying to appease the people who didn't. Although it was easier said than done to shrug off the fact that certain people didn't like me, knowing I had people who did always helped me in my war with worry.

Aside from attempting to scroll on Instagram when #InstagramDown is trending on Twitter, there are few things as pointless as agonising over how much you are liked or disliked. Really, *who cares* if Sarah from uni thinks you're a bit annoying because you put your hand up several times in a lecture? Or if Leyla in marketing doesn't like your latest haircut?

. . . AND BEING LIKED ONLINE

Though it's definitely heightened by social media, being a people pleaser is something that generally carries across from real life into our online presence. The only difference is that online you're not solely trying to keep your mum, best friend, colleague and boss happy, but hundreds or thousands of people at any one time. The thought alone can be overwhelming.

What is more important to you: being liked
in person or being liked online?

In person: 95% | Online: <1% | Don't know: 4%

For years I was worried about being disliked online and, if I'm brutally honest, I probably still am. Only recently have I realised how much time I've spent diluting my opinions, beliefs and thoughts for fear of being 'wrong', or (what feels even worse, in my opinion) disliked. Engaging with others on the internet can sometimes feel like a popularity contest, and we often end up watering down the conversations we'd have confidently with friends in private, in order to appease the masses. This can leave us feeling wishy-washy and incapable of taking a real stance on anything, in case we're perceived as 'too this' or 'too that'. Working online, the desire to adapt ourselves to meet the needs and expectations of strangers can be too much. It's like giving a presentation in front of a thousand random people and hoping that every single one of them is satisfied by what you've said – it's impossible. It's easier to coat ourselves in a metaphorical vanilla flavouring to make sure that we agree with everyone – but all that does is file away the best bits of us. The things that make us unique. The edges we have that nobody else does.

. . . .

'I put so much pressure on myself to achieve, achieve, achieve, but being kind to those who surround you and having that close network is all that really matters.'

AMY, Glasgow

. . . .

YOU CAN BE THE JUICIEST PEACH . . .

. . . but there will always be someone that doesn't like peaches.

It's the 'live, laugh, love!' of friendship advice, but doesn't it ring true? I'm married to a man *who doesn't like Victoria sponge*, for goodness' sake. There are some things that people just don't like – and sometimes it'll be you. A warm, fluffy, oozing-with-jam, homemade-with-love cake that they just can't stomach. But that's fine; look how well the good ol' Viccy sponge is doing! Does it really need another fan? All the more for you, I say.

You can do whatever you like within your power, but there'll always be one person who won't be totally happy. I've heard someone referred to as being 'too nice' before, which assured me that you really can't please all the people

122

all of the time. Just being you – strawberry jam and all – is the best way forward.

#HUMBLEBRAG, #SELFPROMO
OR #BLESSED?

Constant worrying and fretting can leak into moments of success too. The fear of looking like you're bragging is something that steers us away from sharing so much – which, although sometimes a good thing, can also prevent us from moving forward. It's not a quality to be proud of, but knowing the difference between a gentle bit of celebration or self-promotion and a public gluttonous gloat is crucial – and you might be surprised to hear that most people can spot the difference a mile off.

> **Do you ever struggle to talk about your own personal successes?**
>
> Yes: 80% | No: 15% | Don't know: 5%

In work and creative endeavours, self-promotion often comes as part of the job description. If you don't share your work, chances are people are less likely to stumble across it. I know from experience that self-deprecation might seem like the modest answer, but sometimes it's received as a lack of ability and confidence, which contrarily can put people off – typical. It's like we're shooting ourselves in the foot when opportunity knocks, just in case it comes across wrong in the bigger picture. *Psychology of Women Quarterly* published a study stating that 'within American gender norms is the expectation that women should be modest', and that women who violate this 'modesty norm' are conditioned to feel uncomfortable about the prospect of self-promotion.[24] Alice, a member of The Insecure Girls' Club from Manchester, agrees: 'I don't celebrate things enough and I'm constantly looking towards the future/ what I can create next. I'm trying to teach myself to slow down when it matters and to just "sit comfortably" in those periods of success for a little longer.'

Women shouldn't feel that they can't celebrate their successes, nor should modesty be muddled with some healthy self-congratulation – especially in an age where we shouldn't wait for someone else to praise us before we do it ourselves. It's easy to say you've 'just' been working on something you're incredibly proud of, or that it's 'nothing' – but knowing when to throw in a champagne-popping emoji and big yourself up can help other people believe in you, and give yourself that leg up you've been working towards.

'But do you think I offended her?'

. . . .

'Last year I had a mentor at work – she worked with me to realise many things but one particularly stuck out for me. That I didn't celebrate my own achievements and that this was bad for my mental health. I would come into work, think and type as fast as my fingers could go, get the task out of the door and move on to the next one. I realised that I was literally living as a machine. I made the decision to stop and think about what I had achieved at the end of each day. My mentor gave me a notebook for me to write down how I felt on a Monday evening, which really helped me have purpose and to take stock. At the end of the month, she would make me think about what I'd achieved and then ask me how I was going to celebrate that success. I felt such pride in myself that I would never have felt before. The biggest challenge was writing my end-of-year review. Had I not done this work weekly/monthly, I wouldn't have been able to remember what I'd achieved over the course of the year.'

LUCY, London

. . . .

It's the people in life that want you to succeed and care about you the most who will be ready and waiting to cheer you on when you do finally upload that status – and isn't that what matters the most?

LET'S RECAP!

··

From getting red-faced worrying about who we gave the wrong first impression to (I promise she didn't mind you asking where her dress was from), to second-guessing our own opinions and judgements whilst surrounded by those who seem to know their own minds, wondering if we really do need to master the #humblebrag and fretting over unanswered messages on our favourite love-to-hate social media sites – learning to hush the negative monologue that comes with the new and unknown is the first step to doing a Taylor and shakin' it off.

STOP RIGHT NOW,
THANK YOU VERY MUCH

Right! So we've got this far – but how do we stop worrying after meeting new people and going to big events? Is there a way to reclaim power over the small comments we hold on to like hot stones? And how can we put our best thought forward without worrying if we'll mess up?

'But do you think I offended her?'

HALVE THAT PROBLEM!

When I've had moments of pure over-thinking and analysing something to no end, speaking to a friend, explaining the situation and gaining another perspective is one of the most freeing things you can do. Saying it out loud and airing your insecurities can be the first step to whittling down these moments of worry. Nothing makes me feel saner than when I just admit how I've been feeling.

. . . .

'Worrying days, troubled thoughts, tummy-churning moments are still there, I still on occasions feel like that little girl in the playground, but I've learnt to speak about my fears, to share troubles with really good friends, and in that way I hope that I too can be an ear to others. Talking with others and opening up the insecurity conversation is something we must all continue to support.'

CAROLINE, Hertfordshire

. . . .

Call a friend, your mum, or share it on a social media platform and then let the wave of other women who feel the same rush in. Put yourself in the company of people who know you as well as you know yourself and who have your best interests at heart. Often, they've been in the same boat and can realign your worries with a quick phone call or chat. Chances are you'll realise that the person you're fretting over isn't thinking about what *you* said last month because they're too concerned with what *they* said. No one will ever think about you as much as you do, and there's something incredibly reassuring about that.

WHAT IF I'M STILL WORRIED ABOUT THAT UNANSWERED TEXT?

If you're truly concerned about a friendship, try and spark up a gentle conversation or talk about how you're feeling. For example, if you phone and they miss the call, perhaps text a 'Hey! Just phoning for a quick catch-up' to let them know you fancied a chat. However, if it's a little more urgent, perhaps say, 'I've had a bit of a rubbish day – do you have time for a chat?' so they know it's more important and should phone back. Communication is essential, so be honest, but give friends the benefit of the doubt too – not everyone is out to ignore you, I promise.

What we say *vs* what we should say

Oh my God, I did not stop talking at people this evening. Everyone will think I'm so annoying. AND THE JOKES. Oh, the jokes.
I can't believe I chatted to so many new people this evening. I didn't stop talking! I got along with a few ladies, which was nice. I'm so proud of how confident I felt.

I can't believe she's read both of my messages and hasn't replied. I don't know what I've done wrong.
I know she's been really busy with things, so maybe that's why she's not replied to my messages. I'll give her a few days, and if she still hasn't replied I'll give her a ring and check she's OK. You never know what someone else is going through.

I don't agree with what she's said, but I'm worried I'll make a complete tit of myself if I voice my opinion.
I think I'm going to have a chat with her as I've got a different point of view. I don't know everything, but I guess having a discussion can only help to inform my opinion.

Argh, if I share this post about my new job people are going to think I'm so braggy.
I got the job! I'm so proud of myself – I've worked so hard. I'm going to share it online, and not spare a thought for anyone that doesn't like it. I never share things and I GOT THE JOB!

IDENTIFY WHEN WORRY STRIKES

Knowing what the common denominator is for this negative chatter is the key to ensuring we're armed when we know it's going to come out and play. It can be hard to figure out what the link might be, but I find it helps to keep a journal for a month, or add it to the calendar in my phone, in order to narrow it down. Note all the situations where you feel your insecurity or worries are getting the better of you, and flick back to see what you were doing then. Include any alcohol/drugs/medication/PMS too, as they all have such an impact on how you're feeling. Sometimes, when I'm completely overwhelmed by worry, I'll check my period tracker app and find out that it's a timely 'coincidence' – very handy indeed.

PLAN AND PREVENT

Once you've figured out what triggers your inner worrier – for example, you might identify socialising as the common denominator in the situations where you find yourself the most insecure – dig deeper. Do you feel most anxious when you're:

- *Socialising* – meeting up with people who you know?
- *Socialising outside your comfort zone* – meeting new people in a new place, or going out with no set plans?
- *Socialising when you're feeling vulnerable* – meeting up with people when you're already feeling a bit wobbly?

If you can identify the precise pattern, you can prepare for every similar situation: before, during and after. Think about what specifically you find hard in the situation, and the things that *are* in your control. For example:

- *Before* – If you're heading to a party where you won't know many people, get ready with a friend and let them know how you're feeling, or ask to bring someone else along with you if you're going alone. Know that you don't always *have* to leave your comfort zone, and you can always put in some cushioning to make it more bearable – there's no shame in that.
- *During* – Don't be afraid to be honest. If you're feeling worried and you need to step away, go outside for some air, leave early or even confide in someone – do it! In general, openness is met with openness, and sharing

131

something with somebody can relax your mind when it feels like it's running at 100 mph. Also, nobody will mind as much as you think they will. You're not a nuisance.

- *After* – Over time I've picked up techniques that have helped me press mute on the thoughts that pop up on the train home. The quiet moments in the cab (where I'm definitely pretending to be in a music video) that are so often nosily interrupted with self-doubt. If this gal is able to exchange negative back-chat for my favourite hits on Spotify, with a bit of practice I think you can too.

My best advice (as someone who has wasted *hours* attempting to get their inner worrier under control) is to busy your mind with other things. Here are some of my top tips:

- If you know you're going to come out of a party and turn on the worry, make sure you give yourself something else to focus on. Download a podcast with some familiar friendly voices for the way home, bang on your favourite playlist, or phone a friend for a reassuring chat.
- Count your breaths. Download an app like Calm, and indulge in some meditation (or just a bit of Stephen Fry reading to you, which is equally soothing).
- Pack a book. Make sure your journey home is

filled with the story of someone else's life, and not worries about your own.

- People watch! It can be as deep or shallow as you want it to be, but sometimes focusing on others' lives going by offers a sense of perspective when things feel overwhelming.

JUST SAY NO, THANK YOU

If you're going out when you're already feeling wobbly, be honest. Let the people you're meant to be going out with know how you're feeling (even if you'd rather them not mention it when you get there) or simply tell them you're not up to the chase.

I remember an evening last year when I felt stressed to the point of snorty, snotty tears and knew I had a list as long as my arm to do – and a dinner to attend. I was in a bit of a state, but the idea of cancelling made me feel even worse; the stress of having to text and then worry if the host would be angry was just as bad. I was in no shape to get dressed up, let alone leave the house. But after sending a message (and a bunch of flowers to apologise), it felt like a small weight had been lifted. There's no defeat in listening to yourself and taking an evening in when you're not feeling up to it. We're told that it's terrible to cancel plans, and although I try to avoid it whenever possible, if I know I won't be brilliant company (and that going will make me more stressed) then being honest and kind is the best way to go.

USE YOUR 'WEAKNESS' AS YOUR POWER

The traits we fret about can also be reframed as something to be proud of.

. . . .

'Nearly eight years ago, when I met a close friend of my fiancé's she made a comment that stuck with me. Clearly it really hurt me as I still think of it now, nearly eight years on! She said that she thought I tried too hard. Initially I was really upset by this and couldn't stop thinking about it. I obsessed over what exactly she had meant by the comment. I really hate it when people don't like me, so this made me feel even worse. Anyway, I finally realised something – not everyone will like you, not everyone needs to like you, you can't be friends with everyone you meet. And you know what? That took a long time to sink in. I also came to the conclusion that it's OK to "try too hard" – it's great to throw yourself at life, to be enthusiastic, to really show your emotions.'

ABBIE, *London*

. . . .

The worry of being seen as 'attention seeking' when hogging the microphone at karaoke (ahem) can be flipped to make you the 'life and soul of the party', and all those times you've worried you've been fussing over a friend or 'getting on their nerves' are often an indicator of the caring traits you possess. Being one thing to somebody is being something else entirely to another person – you just can't be everything to everyone. Self-awareness isn't a bad thing, but sabotaging your every move with negative back-chat is – so try and flip things around the other way.

If you're struggling to pick things out about yourself that make you the wonderful person you are, speak to someone you trust. Perhaps you've got a friend or family member whose opinion you value. Ask them to give you three things they admire or like about you – write them down, and keep them with you. If you really want to push yourself, recite them in the mirror each day. It might feel a bit ridiculous (especially if you're not used to giving yourself praise), but repeat them and pull them out whenever self-sabotage threatens.

To help you get started, here are some of my favourite positive words and traits. Pick the ones that you relate to (or make someone else pick for you)!
- Funny
- Kind
- Caring

- Thoughtful
- Considerate
- Generous
- Selfless
- Smart
- Quick-witted
- Intelligent
- Brave
- A good listener
- Supportive
- Loving
- Fun
- Friendly
- Creative
- Warm
- Patient
- Cheerful
- A ray of sunshine
- Inspiring

ACCEPT YOU WON'T ALWAYS KNOW THE ANSWERS TO EVERYTHING

And not only is that fine, but it's normal. If we all had everything figured out and never felt compelled to learn, discuss and shape the way we view the world, how dull would that be? If everyone knew everything we'd all be pretty much the same. Accept that we don't have to get everything right first time, you're allowed to change your opinion on things and that sometimes just being part of the conversation is a brilliant and freeing first step. You're not the same person you were five years ago, and every day is an opportunity to learn – so don't let the fear of getting something wrong, or doing something imperfectly, stop you from trying. My brother is an amazing example of this. He's never afraid to start something new with no experience, and in the last few months has invested in a keyboard, kung-fu lessons, and still has a curiosity to try more. He doesn't care about getting it wrong, which is so admirable when getting started can be the scariest thing.

It's important to make mistakes, so having patience with yourself is key. Here are some steps towards that:

- If you get something wrong first time, allow yourself to get frustrated, but don't let it stop you trying again. Look at Edison with the light bulb! It took him 1000 attempts (or 'a 1000-step process' as he said), and look at the pay-off – BULBS!
- Try and remind yourself that you are constantly learning, and being brave enough to try something in the first place is a feat in itself. You have already learnt something from trying.

- If you find yourself getting annoyed, step away from what you're doing and then come back. Take deep breaths and recognise that most things take time – whether you're tackling the full run of *Friends* or writing an essay, it's a process. You don't have to be doing something all hours of the day either – sometimes a few concentrated hours is better than lengthy days filled with procrastination.

- Deal with the situation as if you were a teacher talking to a pupil – they'd have patience with you, and encourage you to take it slowly. Do the same for yourself.

And remember – you can never improve at anything if you don't start in the first place.

Equally, if the idea of getting into a debate brings you out in hives, don't feel you need to always have an opinion or get involved in the first instance. Sometimes the thought of being outspoken and vulnerable brings more stress than the actual conversation itself, and sometimes remaining in your comfort zone is perfectly fine. If you do want to assert yourself, however, learning to trust your gut and own your opinion, even if it's not fully formed, is a powerful tool. Often it isn't really about what you know but the confidence you have whilst saying it – as long as you're willing to learn, and participate in a two-way conversation.

'But do you think I offended her?'

EXIT THE ECHO CHAMBER

We might not have the answers to everything, but broadening our horizons on the net ain't always a bad thing. When elections, polls and results shows haven't 'gone my way', it's made me think a lot about the echo chambers we subconsciously enter online. Being surrounded by similar voices that align with your views and beliefs can make it easy to forget that there are people in the world who share different standpoints – contrasting, conflicted and powerful.

Naturally, online we're prone to following people we gravitate towards – for their music tastes, shopping skills, political views, or ability to tell a side-splitting joke in 140 characters or less. But this can make it difficult for us to understand points of views that are vastly different from our own – and seeing beyond that bubble is integral for self-education, and to mould the way we engage with others who don't feel the same as us. By curating our feeds (perhaps subliminally) this way, we are limiting what we see, and thereby cutting ourselves off from the conversations we should be having with those who aren't in our immediate circles.

If you feel like your views on a topic are a bit one-sided, click on a hashtag, read the comments below a post, or Google reliable sources to build up a more rounded perspective. Make sure your feeds are peppered with people who share different stories to yours. This doesn't mean

139

you have to follow people with completely adverse opin-ions, but not following exclusively the same types of people will allow you to discover new things – whether that's a new band, brand or viewpoint. Kio Stark, author of *When Strangers Meet*, described in her 2016 TED talk how pos-itive interactions with people from different social groups can help eradicate bias and prejudice.[25]

SHARE YOUR SUCCESSES

I've always worried that on Instagram my job, and what I post about, comes across as 'The Liv Show'. That people are sitting on their phones, eyes rolling, going, 'Oh, not again!' when a picture I post pops up, or when I share the link to a blog post I've been working on. But, thinking about it, isn't that what Instagram is for? Of course it's going to be 'The Liv Show', because it's my personal account. If you don't want to see me, then why on earth are you here, pal? Real-ising that the people that follow you are largely rooting for your successes should hopefully mean that you are able to root for your successes too – and hey, if they aren't, are they really the kind of people you want to be following you in the first place? Obviously, balancing out self-promotion (which should always be shameless, FYI) with different facets of your life online is important, but by being tact-ful with our timing and owning the moment, we should always feel proud enough to share our achievements when they arise. And this doesn't have to be solely online: if you hand in a huge piece of coursework, get a new job or make it through a probation period, take your celebration into the real world.

> You could:
> - Go for a drink after work.
> - Phone up your friend and suggest dinner out or a takeaway.
> - Watch your favourite film and have a solo pamper evening.
> - Plan a fun day with your best friend when you're both next free.
> - Treat yourself to something you've been saving up for, or waiting for.
> - Text your nearest and dearest the good news (they'll be glad you did).

Sharing and celebrating the small successes in life and realising it's OK to be your own spokesperson really is the key to some serious self-validation.

Sarah Powell

podcast host, columnist and founder of Celebrate Yourself

Having started her wonderful business, Celebrate Yourself (offering wedding ceremonies and courses on self-celebration), after some time feeling a little lost, Sarah knows what it feels like to worry about which direction you're going in and pleasing those around you. An online (and off) ray of sunshine, she shares her tips on celebrating yourself and putting your worries to one side.

Sarah, you're one of my favourite people to follow online for many reasons. You talk so candidly about everything from confidence to body image and being enough – where did it all begin, and how did you become so comfortable opening up online about all of life's little wobbles?

It all began when my full-time radio show ended. I was at home with no one to talk to or connect with, so I started chatting away on Instagram stories. Most of my followers at that point were people I knew, so I just imagined chatting to my friends. I would talk about the most mundane everyday stuff. And then new people began to join in, and the lovely thing was that people recognised themselves in what I was talking about. I started talking about my insecurities and anxiety and body confidence issues, and people sent me messages saying 'me too!' and thanking me for sharing. It felt really lovely to know I wasn't alone with how I was feeling. It has now become the most gorgeous support network; I feel like complete strangers online are my friends because I chat to them every day. I need the support and sharing as much as they do because we're all in this together.

You've spoken before about the anxiety that came with wanting to be liked by everyone – which is something I know so many of us experience. How did you bring that worrying to a halt and manage your own expectations, as well as those of others?
My whole life I have always been a people pleaser and desperate to be liked. I really believed that if I could be liked, everything would be OK. I would always place everyone's opinion of me before my own and spent hours worrying what people thought of me. It was very crippling and confusing and gave me a lot of anxiety.

When the radio show finished and I was in the wilderness, I made a decision to change and I knew the people pleasing had to go. I told myself, 'I am a good person who is trying my best,' and if other people didn't like me that was OK, because I like me. So I made the switch from worrying about what other people thought about me to what I thought about me, which I know sounds simple but it really worked. The relief of letting go was huge and now I'm so much more calm and confident.

I think it's also really important to remember that doing

something new, in front of new people or strangers, is going to make you feel vulnerable. It's those moments when we really need to be kind to ourselves and find our self-compassion, and lean a bit more on the people we love rather than needing everyone to give their approval.

The big one! Is there a way we can accept we won't be liked by everyone? It sounds silly, but I think we really struggle to accept that some people won't like us, despite how hard we try. It's a daunting prospect!
It *is* daunting! And a few years ago I would never have been able to contemplate that some people wouldn't like me. It would have worried me to death and made me super anxious. Placing so much importance on other people liking you means you lose a lot of power, because your self-worth is dictated by them and not you.

I read something which really helped me: what other people think of you is none of your business. I know this might sound harsh but it's completely true. Apart from your close friends and family, you will never know what someone else truly thinks of you. You never know what is going on for someone else and they never know what's going on for you. Especially if it's a stranger online or otherwise. So lay that down. Let it go and save all that energy to like yourself.

Finally, remember *you* don't like everyone. There are some people who get on your wick and others you just don't take to at all, so the same is true of how people feel about you.

If you're feeling a little lost on where to start, what are your top three tips for celebrating yourself?
Babes! I'll go even better and give you five!

- Know that whatever is happening, you are doing your best. You're a work in progress and you aren't expected to have mastered everything right now.
- Accept yourself, exactly as you are right now. However tired, happy, hungry you are. Accept your weight, how you look, how you feel, and everything as you in this moment; then you can decide what to do next.
- Celebrate three tiny wins from today, no matter how small. In fact, the smaller celebrations are often the best ones. Filled up your water bottle? Finished your lunch? Remembered your headphones? Celebrate it, babes.
- Place self-compassion above criticism. Showing yourself kindness is the greatest act of self-love there is. No matter how small.
- Know your worth and show up for it. Say no if you need to, ask for help if you want it, and don't save anything 'for best'. Believe in your worth and other people will too.

You're a podcast host, celebrant, columnist (plus TV and radio presenter) and all-round self-celebration expert – how do you 'put yourself out there' without worrying about what everyone thinks?

I started off small, thinking, 'No one will listen to/read/watch this!' That gave me the comfort and confidence to just relax and have fun. If we overthink things, we get uptight and lose our authenticity, and then it's harder to connect. I also started to believe that my audience would find me. I decided it was better to have a handful of people who loved what I did than to try and please everyone. That was a huge turning point for me. It meant I relaxed and tried new things without worrying too much, and the best thing is that it was those things (my podcast/stories/column) which have connected the most, because I was just being me.

Finally, you're a woman with lots of sunshiny feel-good wisdom – do you have any words of compassion or mantras for members of The Insecure Girls' Club to add to their repertoire?

'I am doing my best.' Please remember that in any given situation, you are always trying your best with however things are right now. Also remember what our saviour RuPaul says: 'If you can't love yourself, how the hell are you going to love someone else?!' You can't give to anyone else if you aren't happy, secure and showing yourself love. And finally, 'More is more.' More eyeliner, more wine, more kindness, more self-celebrations and more love, please.

Takeaway pick-me-ups for silencing negative back-chat, from The Insecure Girls' Club

- Realise most people are as worried about how they come across as you are. You're doing brilliantly – trust me.
- If you can, try not to check your 'read' receipts. People are busy and they don't always realise that they've dropped the ball.
- Accept that we're all a work in progress. Failures are part of the learning curve and our development. Be able to get things wrong, be patient with yourself, and come out the other side with an arsenal of life lessons.
- Trust your gut and own your opinions. If you don't have faith in yourself, then who else will?
- There is nothing wrong with admitting you don't know something. Nobody knows it all. You might be an expert in 2000 number-one pop hits and that's BRILL. Don't worry that you don't have all the other answers.
- The people that care about you are all that matter. Share your new job! Flaunt those wedding photos! The people who love you will want to see you do well and celebrate alongside you.
- If in doubt, air that insecurity! Talk to those who know you well and have your best interests at heart. A problem shared is a problem halved, and if you're worried you've come across a certain way, having someone who knows you better than you know yourself is a sure-fire way to iron out any doubts.

5

'I'm worried they don't like me': forging friendships and maintaining old ones

Ditching people pleasing (mostly)
and navigating friendships

In a lot of ways, friendships are like romantic relationships. Sometimes they start with a hormone-fuelled bang – the hysterical 'I've just met someone who is *basically me*' at school; the burst of excitement at finding someone so akin to you it's like they're your soulmate. Sometimes there are the slow but civilised coffee dates, the back and forth of texts and not knowing where this could go. The 'I saw this and thought of you' messages. They're able to bring you butterflies of excitement after not seeing them for a while, six-pack-inducing laughter, evenings in with tubs of Ben & Jerry's, favourite films and late-night gossiping with in-jokes only the two of you share, adventures abroad, and intimacies revealed that mark the beginning of something special. 'WE'VE HAD THE POO CHAT! THAT'S SAYING SOMETHING!' I mean, *come on*, often romantic partners don't even know the ins and outs of your period cycle and bowel movements – *odd*! Friends really are *something else* – and finding the people or person you feel most comfortable with can rival a love interest ten times over.

I've always said my best friend Gemma is like a soulmate. Because although boys are fun, she's always pretty much been my number one. After finding ourselves next to each other in the register at secondary school (God bless the alphabet and our surnames!), we've laughed together, cried together, tried to hide going to each other's houses after school by getting on separate buses so that people didn't think we were weird together, queued up for gigs in the rain together, survived our first festival together – and walked down the aisle together (albeit not to marry one another).

But like a confusing boyfriend or tricky girlfriend, friendships can bring uncertainty. Messages left unanswered, bickering, fallouts, and different expectations that mean you're not always on the same page. There are long-distance challenges, jealousy, and sometimes things naturally drift their separate ways – sometimes for the worst but often for the best.

As I've got older I've become more able to identify the different kinds of friends we develop in life. Growing up surrounded by strong female groups, I've been fortunate enough to see the qualities of hardy friendships, but having also been a hormonal teenager fuelled on tears, a Panic! At The Disco obsession and lots of confusion, I know what it's like to feel at a total loss with friendships – wondering what you've done wrong if someone goes off-grid and pondering how to repair a bond when it's only you fighting for it. There are so many different threads of insecurity that feed into modern female friendship. We've all worried about whether we've been a good enough friend; whether we're supportive, available and reliable enough. Do I make enough time for my friends? Am I trying too hard with her? Does she want to hang out with me? Am I even capable of making new friends? It doesn't matter whether you're thinking about new relationships or old: we're all prone to moments of self-doubt over our friendships (as well as juggling all our other concerns).

THE NATURAL EVOLUTION OF FRIENDSHIPS (SAID IN YOUR FINEST DAVID ATTENBOROUGH VOICE)

From all-girls-school bitchiness to first boyfriends (I remember feeling like I'd been replaced in a heartbeat when my best friend got her first boyfriend – incredibly melodramatic considering I had my own boyfriend), from relocating to making friends as a grown-up, friendships naturally morph with time.

> **How long have you known your best friends for?**
>
> 1–2 years: 4% | 3–6 years: 27% | 7+ years: 66% | Don't know: 2% | Prefer not to say: 1%

What with work, family life and the banalities of the day-to-day, friendship goes from being something organically embedded into each day at school to something we have to make time for. We're no longer sitting next to our best friend every day at a desk, and in the modern world – due to higher education, new jobs, new partners and families – we're further away from the people we grew up with than ever before. More hurdles pop up, and sometimes getting a date in the diary with your best friend feels like completing a level in a video game. It can be incredibly difficult to navigate, and the transition from seeing your friends every day to perhaps once a month can often leave you feeling secondary – a strange reality if you're used to being in each other's pockets.

Expectations in a friendship will also shift as life changes. Lauren, a member of The Insecure Girls' Club from London, says, 'I get very jealous of my mates having other mates – I never say anything but it must stem from being younger. I know it's me feeling insecure that I'm not wanted any more, which is so untrue but it's inside me.' Friendships will experience growing pains, and taking these into consideration is part of nourishing a healthy friendship. It's the way you adjust and communicate that matters; being able to understand that although you both have new commitments and priorities, it doesn't mean you don't care for each other the way you did when you were spending every day together. It's the same relationship, just with the extra embellishments and threads of adulthood woven through.

In our teens and into our twenties, friendships can also become like fast fashion. Instead of maintaining and looking after relationships that fill us up and offer us something meaningful and, for want of a better word, useful, we can find ourselves flitting around new people, drawn to the excitement of the unknown and forgetting about the bricks-and-mortar relationships that age as well as a brilliant Breton T-shirt compared to a sequinned neon Topshop piece. The buzz of making a new friend can feel heady and exciting, and sometimes we can end up 'collecting' new friends instead of looking at what we already have (a little like clothes shopping). A 2009 study by Dutch sociologist Gerald Mollenhorst found that as we get older a lot of our friendships will evolve and change, with new friends replacing older ones and most close friendships only lasting seven years – showing that nurturing the ones we care about is integral to their longevity.[26]

> **Have you made a new best friend over the age of twenty-one?**
>
> Yes: 48% | No: 45% | Don't know: 5% | Prefer not to say: 2%

LITTLE FRIENDS AND BIG FRIENDS

As someone who returned from my summer holiday to Spain in Year 6 armed with beaded friendship bracelets and strips of Looney Tunes sweets from the shop that sold sun cream – and a Post-it note on everything to catch up on when school started again in September, it's safe to say I have always been excited by friendships. But as we get older, our friendships become woven with more complexity than whether we brought the right colour friendship band back from holiday. Even if our friendships are of equal value, some will work vastly differently from others, and sometimes navigating them well can be a learning curve. One friend might be the kind you share dinner with every six months, another an accomplice on your daily commute, but if they're not the kind that require intense text-tennis every day, it doesn't mean they're not important.

As humans, we crave company, and it can feel like second nature to desire additional friendships and 'grow' our circle.

. . . .

'Recently, I stopped craving friendships. I've decided that friendships will happen when they do. People come into your life for different reasons. Some come to make you smile on your trip to the supermarket, some to hang out all summer at the beach, and some to become your lifelong friends. And that's OK.'

CHRISTINA, *New York*

. . . .

To me, a longing for friendship is linked to a longing for connection – and whilst our friendship groups may not look how we think they 'should' all the time, we are presented with opportunities to connect with people every day, so an open mind can be invaluable (even if it does take a little bravery).

How to find sparks of connection in your day-to-day:

- Compliment someone on their outfit. Seen someone wearing those & Other Stories heels you've been lusting over? Go forth and tell them how great they look!
- Spotted someone reading a book by your favou-

rite author? Tell them how much you love them too, and ask how they're finding it.

- Go for a walk around the park after work, and say hello to someone you pass. I find a park (even if you don't have a dog) is a place where (most) people are happy to say hello, and sometimes even have a natter.

- If you catch a bus to work or school, there's always an opportunity to chat to the person next to you if something connects you (be it an article they're reading or a moment you share). This is possibly the scariest one of them all, but sometimes just getting on and sitting down when it's pouring with rain outside can be the moment to say, 'Can you believe this weather?!'

- Try chatting to someone in the queue at the supermarket – they don't have to be your soulmate, but sometimes a small interaction can lift you when you need it. Ask the cashier how their day is going. I once sat outside Sainsbury's with my dog whilst waiting for someone inside, and ended up talking to the security guard for half an hour. We spoke about her husband and her daughters, and although I haven't seen her since, it was nice to chat to someone and share the everyday.

ON LONELINESS AND MAKING
NEW FRIENDS

I don't think loneliness is ever something you factor in when you think of friendship in early adulthood. The term alone conjures up images of an old-age pensioner, with her lilac rinse and rollers in, looking out of a rain-soaked window, waiting for her family to pop by on a Sunday afternoon. Not a twenty-something PhD student feeling at a loss for what to do on a Friday night. It's one of the hardest feelings to admit to – and, much like pubic hair, your salary and your thoughts on Brexit, it feels strangely taboo for something we all experience at one point or another. With one in three 18–24-year-olds feeling lonely compared to one in ten 64–72-year-olds (according to a survey conducted by the Young Women's Trust in 2018),[27] it's something that affects more of us than we probably realise. But surprisingly (or not), a full WhatsApp inbox and an Instagram bursting with comments don't always mean you won't experience loneliness. For some, social media might satisfy their sociable fix, but it's important to identify the kind of interaction that works best for you, to keep any feelings of isolation at bay.

Have you ever struggled making friends?

'I struggle to find the balance between knowing when to text or not. And when I meet people through other friends I feel like I can't message them without including the original friend, which makes it hard to expand your circle.'   *Emma, London*

It's easy to look inwards when it comes to feeling lonely, too; assuming we're to blame for feeling like this.

. . . .

'I think it's something that so many people don't think they can discuss, if they're feeling a bit lonely without thinking they sound like a bit of a loser, especially when everyone on social media/celebs are always talking about their "girl squadz". Growing apart from old school friends, moving away from your hometown or starting new jobs can be so daunting and isolating.'

EMMA, *Manchester*

. . . .

The pressure to have a Taylor Swift-style 'girl squad' can certainly be overwhelming. With many brands now parading #SquadGoals and #GirlGangs in their ads, if you don't have your squad 'sorted' it can feel isolating, especially when all you want is someone to chat with about the latest Louis Theroux documentary. As positive as those intentions may be, having a solid, big set of girlfriends (who, if you're judging by the adverts, all wear girl-band matching clothes) is simply unrealistic. It takes away from the truth of quality over quantity; if I've learnt anything about friendships whilst growing up, it's not the number you have but the quality of the few you have that matters. Take the pressure off yourself and start small. Friendships grow where you water them, and if you have a garden as big as a festival field, chances are their quality won't be as good.

FRIENDS WITH COMMON GROUND

There will be a handful of times in life when you'll be in the exact same position as others when it comes to making friends, and this is a prime time to make the most of it; whether it's having a new next-door neighbour, or a new roommate at university.

. . . .

'Making friends as an adult is hard! I meet so many great people through friends, or through work – but then actually meeting up with them outside that context is a whole different thing. I'd be scared that they would pie me off, it's like when you start seeing a new boy and you're scared they'll go off you!'

CHLOE, *London*

. . . .

When I had just moved up to Liverpool for university, every time someone told me, 'Oh, don't be scared, you're all in the same boat,' I could feel my eyes rolling. 'Sure, but that doesn't make it any less scary,' I'd think, watching people walk into lectures, looking out for a familiar band T-shirt, a look of nervousness or simply a sign they'd want to be friends with me. But it's true – although I went to as many freshers' nights as I could count on one hand, everyone was happy to chat if I mumbled my way up to them, because at the end of the day, who doesn't want a new pal? Plus, vulnerability is usually met with kindness and a reciprocal openness – especially if the vulnerability you're revealing is mutual. All it takes is one person to make the difficult first move – and whoever does it, you can guarantee it'll be appreciated. Whether you're starting at somewhere new for work, joining a new mums' group, or even striking up a conversation with the fellow student or freelancer who perches in the same cafe spot as you every day, it's always worth it.

FRIENDSHIP BREAK-UPS

On the other hand, the one thing that never gets easier with age is a grotty friendship break-up.

Have you ever had a friendship break-up?

'After six years. It genuinely felt like heartbreak and was a friendship break-up that I didn't see coming, nor understand why it was happening (and it was by text!).'

Emily, Maidenhead

I used to, and in fact still do, find friendship break-ups one of the most confusing things *ever*. Friendships are meant to be the easier, more relaxed and less daunting version of a romantic relationship – so why do things like this happen? It's so hard when someone you considered close begins ghosting you or changing the way they treat you, with text replies becoming few and far between, and a growing sense of discomfort replacing carefree chatter and laughter.

There's rarely a slamming match or screaming argument that ends a friendship, and sometimes it's the silence and lack of closure that makes a friendship break-up so hard to let go of. When it's happened to me in the past (for reasons I still don't know), I've felt endless anxiety about it for years because I've let the worry plague me, and every time that person pops up in conversation I'm left wondering what happened. I've imagined a parallel universe where I could confront a friend in confidence – asking them what happened, or what I did wrong, and allowing the situation to come to an end in a healthy, clear-cut way.

Unfortunately not every friendship will last forever and, as with ill-fated romantic relationships, that's fine. Friendships can be there for a reason, a season or a lifetime (as a wise anonymous someone once said). I like to think you can learn a lesson from most things in life, and even if a friendship isn't forever, you'll hopefully be able to take something away from it, no matter how difficult it might feel at the time.

LETTING GO OF TOXIC PALS

When is the right moment to call time on a friendship and start weaning someone out of your life? How do you spot the signs that it's best to go your separate ways? Identifying a toxic friendship isn't always easy, but knowing you feel bad in the company of someone who's supposed to be your mate is a pretty telling sign that things aren't going well. They don't need to have kicked your cat or deleted your series link to *Blue Planet* to prove they shouldn't be in your good books. In general, a friendship isn't meant to fill you with worry, anxiety or uncertainty. It's not supposed to make you feel annoying, bad about yourself, or to damage your confidence. If you come away from seeing someone feeling worse than before you met up, and if someone is only there for you when they need something, perhaps it's worth having a word with yourself about how valuable to your happiness they truly are.

. . . .

'Personally, I've always found friendship quite difficult. I've had several bad experiences in which I felt so out of place with the people around me. I stress the importance of surrounding yourself with people that make you happy, that make you laugh, that make you feel good about yourself. There's absolutely no point in hanging around people that make you feel inferior to them or unworthy. Trust me, as a teenage girl I know. You might find that you don't necessarily like the people that surround you, but feel like if you let them go, you'll have no one. That is OK, though. It's so much better being alone and not being surrounded by negativity than hanging out with people that make you feel unhappy.'

AMELIA, *Australia*

. . . .

And really, I think that's the reason so many of us are scared to let bad friendships go. If your confidence has been knocked, it can feel like you won't meet another friend that can fill their place again. But having a little friendship-shaped hole in your life left by someone who didn't treat you properly is always preferable to being filled up with worries that leave you feeling 'less than'.

It's also worth noting that if a friend isn't there for you on one occasion, it doesn't mean they won't be there next time. You don't have to ditch people that don't support your every move, and giving someone the benefit of the doubt is always beneficial if it's a friendship you truly value. If you love them, you don't have to let them go at the first hurdle – just don't make them top of your priority list. Second chances are there for a reason, and some friends will be better at certain times than others – but just be aware when things become one-sided.

MANAGING EXPECTATIONS

Much like the plants in your garden (or the succulents in your bathroom), not every friendship will require the same amount of TLC. Some don't need much watering at all to survive, while others are like the vase of flowers that need their water changing every three days. The expectations of every friendship are different, but it's essential to be able to manage those expectations with one another. For example, as I mentioned in Chapter 4, I am renowned for being useless over text and WhatsApp: I find responding to endless messages completely overwhelming. Some friends understand

and take it with a pinch of salt (expectation managed), but others may see it as rude – and I've found the expectation to be available at all times considerably challenging. Fortunately (or not), I'm not the only one: research conducted by the Royal Bank of Scotland found that 'one in four young people admit to struggling to respond to calls, texts and social media notifications' and 'a quarter of 18–24-year-olds said they found the pressure difficult to manage' – showing that it's normal to feel like it's hard to switch off.[28]

If you've read *The Five Love Languages* by Gary Chapman, you'll know that in a relationship there are essentially five ways to 'express and experience love', known as the 'love languages'. These include: words of affirmation (kind words to build up the other person), gifts, acts of service, quality time and physical touch.[29] I believe we can transfer this concept to friendships; even if you're a terrible texter like me, I'm sure you have other qualities that make you a great friend, whether that's always remembering birthdays, being in charge of a brilliant get-together, or even just delivering a bloody good hug when it's needed. There might be pressure to be all of these things at the same time, but remember to note the qualities you do possess that make you the friend you are. We all nurture friendships differently, and that's OK.

PEOPLE (AHEM, PAL) PLEASING

From struggling to organise a birthday meal because you're busy thinking of absolutely everyone's dietary requirements other than your own, to feeling responsible for everyone's happiness and wellbeing above yours; from not sharing your problems because they feel like a burden on others, to wanting to be the good guy and agreeing to do something just because it'll make someone else happy – people pleasing is something most of us probably do without even realising. It doesn't mean you have an ulterior motive or are secretly point scoring: some of us (slowly raises hand) simply can't help it. People pleasing within friendships is a difficult line to tread, and getting the balance right between keeping others happy and maintaining your own happiness is key. But people pleasing in friendships can feel harder than people pleasing in general. With friendships, you're not just appeasing someone you barely know to keep up appearances, but because you genuinely care about them and feel invested in keeping them happy.

So, when is the line crossed? Is running the risk of burnout worth it to keep others chipper? And when is it OK not to people please?

When it's OK to do it . . .

Sometimes, saying yes when you'd rather not has to be done. The act of being selfless is fundamental in any friendship, and recognising when to be there and show up is part of being a good friend. Take a friend's birthday, for example. It's on a Tuesday night (I *know*) in the city centre, and it'll take you over an hour to get there. You've got work the next morning and you won't know anyone else there – but your friend has already had plenty of people cancel. Showing up when it'd be far easier not to is when being a people pleaser can be a brilliant thing – and it shows more signs of being a good friend than it does a pushover.

And when it's best not to . . .

If you find yourself continually bending over backwards for a friend, remembering birthdays, sending cards for every occasion, and pulling favours when they can't so much as reply to a text saying they can't make it, maybe it's time to draw the line. It's important to remember you can still be a nice, decent person and not people please, and you don't have to cut people out because of it either. Knowing that you don't always have to say yes doesn't make you a terrible person.

Often we people please to keep others happy whilst battling an internalised fear of confrontation. Getting on the wrong side of someone can quickly mean that we're *sure* they'll never want to speak to us again, let alone rearrange the dinner we can't make. But it is possible to set your own boundaries and assert yourself without being a stern person. You'll be pleased to know that there's a happy middle ground between sugary-sweet people pleaser and bolshie brash woman willing to walk all over people for her own benefit.

I get it – if, like me, the thought of saying no brings you out in a cold sweat worthy of a lie-down in bed, that's understandable. Going against a natural 'yes, man' reaction isn't easy, but there are ways of politely saying no without starting a *Love Island*-style confrontation. For example, if you apologise all the time, people will assume you need to be apologising and start walking all over you, but if you've acted in a reasonable manner, asserted yourself and someone has still been off with you, that is not your burden to bear. You are not in charge of how other people feel. One of the most important parts of friendship is being open and honest about things – so sending a message or making a call, and then letting it go and moving on, can be the best tactic for the insecure girl. If you are decisive and assertive, that doesn't take away from you being a good, likeable person – it just means you can have a bit of authority over a situation, which is never a bad thing. Amy, a member of The Insecure Girls' Club from London, agrees: 'I've learnt the most important relationship you have is with yourself. I have been running on empty for a long time, trying to be everything to everyone and living up to people's enormous expectations, forgetting about myself in the process.'

If you spend so long obsessing over who might not like what you're doing, you'll never get anything done.

The truth is, we're all just figuring it out as we go. No one is the perfect friend all of the time, and whether you've found your soulmate, your best friend, or just someone to have a coffee with once in a while, navigating any friendship is always a learning curve.

LET'S RECAP!

....

From new friendships to brazen poo chats, private jokes and girlie holidays with old ones, from dealing with breakups and shedding friendships that have gone sour to navigating people pleasing and developing the confidence to shrug off being liked, friendship can require more work than a hefty dissertation. But the pay-off is rewards far greater and longer lasting than a mortarboard hat and a few letters after your name, so it is always worth the perseverance.

STOP RIGHT NOW, THANK YOU VERY MUCH

Looks like we made it! So, how do we maintain the mates we have, cope when things go wrong, and make sure we're able to assert ourselves without worrying about what others think first? You won't be able to win 'em all, but you can learn to focus on what you have and come out the other side if the going gets tough.

FIND THOSE FRIENDS!

When squad goals and loneliness feel overwhelming, the question is, 'How on earth do I find new friends?' If the idea of community service doesn't get you going (a nice and simple Google suggestion when asked 'how to make new friends'), then it's time to look elsewhere. Having recently moved to Brighton from California, Graciela, a member of The Insecure Girls' Club, explains, 'Growing up I struggled to make friends but always managed to find a way. Now though, I don't even know where to start. It makes me feel extremely vulnerable to see that I have to start from scratch. I am nowhere near as cool as the people around me and now I fear it's too late.' It can be palm-sweatingly daunting to approach a random stranger in a coffee shop, so is there any other way to dip your toe into friendship making without breaking out into a hot sweat? Come on – as if being lonely wasn't enough, now I have to be vulnerable too?!

One way to discover new friends is to follow your interests. My other half always says that if he's unwillingly brought along as my 'plus-one' to events, if he has football to chat about he can pretty much talk to anyone, however anxiety-inducing he might find it. Seek out extra-curricular things going on near you. Are you an avid reader? Perhaps there's a book club on your doorstep filled with other people who also felt strongly about Sally Rooney's new novel! As clichéd as it is, giving new things a go can be a win-win too. If you've always craved a bit of pottery action, then perhaps turn the opportunity to do something new into a friendship-making moment – the worst-case scenario is that you don't meet your new BFF but instead come away with a swanky new skill (and a slightly wonky new vase). So many brands are now doing workshops and shopping events; even heading along to something nearby after work could be the start of something beautiful (as well as a chance to utilise that 10 per cent discount code).

Plus, there's THE INTERNET (in the least patronising way possible)! Thankfully, over the last ten years reaching out to a stranger online has become far less taboo (obviously once you've done your precautionary checks and can 100 per cent confirm they are a real human). I remember the fear of telling my mum and dad I'd made some friends on Myspace and wanted to meet up with them. I could see their eyes glaze over with fear that their daughter had made a friend *online*. Thankfully, after meeting them (and my now husband) they're far more amenable to the idea. And with apps like Bumble BFF and Peanut (for mamas) now available, friend dating is even easier. Plus, who said sliding into someone's DMs has to mean romance? If you follow someone – be it a blogger, local florist or just someone with similar interests to you who happens to be nearby – what's the harm in suggesting a coffee? I know I've felt scared at the thought of essentially 'chatting someone up', but if some one asked me for a cuppa and a slice of cake, I definitely couldn't be more chuffed.

KNOW IT'S NEVER TOO LATE FOR A MATE

Throw generation gaps, societal expectations and friendship preconceptions in the recycling bin, and approach making a new friend with no expectations. It's never too late to meet a new friend – and whether you're in your teens or have teenagers of your own, it certainly doesn't mean your friendship quota is up.

. . . .

'For me, working with the elderly and having such close bonds with my grandparents has taught me an awful lot. It taught me about selflessness, it taught me to look after my mental health, and that our elderly generation has so much more to give than any of us can imagine. After I left my role as a physiotherapist specialising in elderly care within the NHS, I suppose I felt a void that I wasn't sure how to fill. I found out about the Age UK Befriending scheme through a friend and immediately signed up. I chose Age UK because they are wildly underfunded, and maybe I could help someone who was lonely? And having an elderly pal was the best thing since sliced bread to me. I was matched with a Northern Irish lady in her nineties and we shared stories over countless cups of tea, spent time in her beautiful garden, and even popped out to the Savoy for a very fancy afternoon tea. She honestly has been a light in my life. She taught me that life is too short to worry over small things, and that whilst your legs work – use them!'

LINDSEY, *London*

. . . .

So, like Lindsey, check out opportunities in your local area. There are meet-ups happening all the time (I found some recently in our local 'zine): checking what's going on locally can be a great starting point.

GIVE YOURSELF A CHANCE!

Try not to expect the worst when making new friends. We can feel overwhelmed when we meet someone new and our inner critic reminds us of the times when we weren't successful, but try and assume the best instead. What if it goes really well? What if you click straight away? What if they say they also have a soft spot for terrible emo bands?

Shift your perspective: if they don't happen to be your soulmate, it doesn't matter. You tried – and each time you try you can know that you've pushed yourself a little out of your comfort zone, which in this case is something to be celebrated and will make it easier next time. Know that you have plenty of things other people are looking for in a friend, and know you're of value to somebody else too.

What we say *vs* what we should say

I'm never going to meet any more friends, this is impossible – HELP ME.
Making new friends is hard – but I've just become a member of a local book club and registered for a few events, so I'm hoping I'll meet some like-minded people there.

Ugh, she's been so useless at texting back – she either doesn't like me or is doing this on purpose.
I've not heard from her in a while, and she's been a bit rubbish with texts. I hope she's OK – maybe I'll check in once more to see if things are all right. You never know what's going on, and being patient and honest is the best way forward.

> *No, I don't mind where we go for dinner this evening.*
> Hey! Have you guys heard about the new Italian down the road? I was thinking we could give that a try?

COPING WITH A FRIENDSHIP BREAK-UP

One of the main reasons friendship break-ups are hard is that the person you're breaking up with is the one you'd probably be venting to on any other occasion. They're the person you'd invite round for a pizza, some ITVBe and a cry – so losing them can feel a whole lot more isolating and difficult to navigate than a romantic break-up.

Instead of getting a dramatic new haircut, perhaps consider doing things to boost yourself if you're feeling low. Allow yourself to wallow for a bit – you're only human – but then pick yourself up and remember to care for yourself as you would anyone else.

Here are some of my favourite ways to pick your-self up (and get yourself back on your feet):

- Go for a run with your favourite podcast in your ears (and when you get home, book tickets to that live podcast event to meet other listeners).
- Consider joining a club – a book club, a life drawing class, a netball team, a tennis club, what-ever! – that will open up new doors and make you feel better about yourself.
- Take a cooking class and get chatting to the person next to you.
- If you're anything like me, write it out. Do a bit of teen-angst journalling and write down all of your feelings so they're somewhere other than in your head.
- Go for after-work drinks with colleagues, and perhaps sit next to someone you haven't chatted to much before.

Finally, if the break-up has happened and you know some-thing you've done has contributed to it, see if you can learn something from it. If you identify bad habits you know you need to work on, maybe it's the perfect time to address them and start afresh. It won't soothe the pain straight away, but knowing you're able to come away a better person eventually might help you find a little solace when things are rocky.

Kate Leaver

journalist and author of
The Friendship Cure

With an archive of agony aunt articles and a book on modern friendships (and how to navigate them), there's not much Kate Leaver doesn't know when it comes to the ups and downs of female friendships. From tackling loneliness to making friends for the first time, we talk about how to embrace being vulnerable (with minimal sweaty-handedness) . . .

Kate, in 2018 you published your debut book *The Friendship Cure*, which covers everything from online friendships and making friends to fallouts, work wives and mental illness. What was the biggest thing you took away from it? I learnt a lot speaking to so many women about modern friendship. I got this very strong sense of how much women mean to each other, what joy and solidarity and loyalty we give each other, and just how powerful our friendships can be. I knew female friendship was this profound and wonderful force, but it was just a joy to prove that to myself by speaking to so many people about it. I also discovered, though, how easily and how ferociously we can tear each other down.

For every story of hope and love and tenderness, I also got one about heartache and betrayal and grief. I wrote a chapter about friendship break-ups and for that, women generously told me about times they were ghosted, lied to, criticised and let down by people they loved. Some of them described a break-up as being like a death, because it really is a form of grief that you go through when someone disappears from your life. That really stayed with me.

I also learnt that loneliness can affect everyone. Even perky twenty-three-year-olds who feel like they don't have anyone to go with them to a Paramore concert. I learnt that it's entirely possible to have and make real, lasting friendships online. I learnt that a lot of us feel lied to by the TV show *Friends* because not everyone gets such a neat, dependable group of friends they see all the time. I learnt that we have a scheduling problem, especially in the UK, and most people are overwhelmed by their diaries, their careers and their expectations of themselves. I learnt that friendship is as important as it's ever been, if not more so.

Following on from that – at any point did it make you realise that no matter how glamorous, organised or successful each of us seems, we all tackle qualms with navigating different friendships?
YES. Truly, no matter how glamorous or put together or ambitious or successful people are, they still seem to struggle with navigating friendship in some way. Even people with very shiny lives have secret fears and qualms and concerns about their friends. Those who seem to have their life utterly together can be lonely, confused, scared of rejection and worried about their friends. Loneliness does not discriminate and

certainly, glamour and success do not make us immune to it. A glossy Instagram profile does not protect us from loneliness, from rejection or from fear. Worrying about your lovability as a person is a very human, very natural thing, and it affects so many people you wouldn't expect. Friendship can be a difficult thing to navigate and maintain – and that goes for everyone.

Loneliness and meeting new people can feel like two pretty taboo topics. Have you experienced it before, and how have you combatted it?
Absolutely, I've been lonely before. I'm yet to speak to some-one who hasn't. I think, to a certain extent, a bit of loneliness is a natural part of the human condition. I think it's a bit out of control now, and it can get chronic and be dangerous for us. I've been lonely because I work at home, so I don't have work colleagues. I've been lonely because I live with depression, and that can be extremely isolating. I have fought it with a delib-erate effort on my part to reconnect with friends. Sometimes, especially when I'm sad, I don't feel like leaving the house and seeing people. I've trained myself to know when I can push past that and see people anyway, and I've also learnt to be comfortable sending little messages to tell people I can't. I'm getting better at telling people when I'm down and asking for support or help, which makes me feel less alone. Also, I got a dog! Which helps enormously with loneliness. He's my little companion while I work, I meet people at the park who talk to me because I have a dog, and I feel less alone because he's always with me. I actually pick up the phone and organise a gentle hang-out with someone I trust and love when I'm feel-ing lonely. I also try and name it – it helps to say out loud or to

myself that I feel lonely because once I've identified what it is, it doesn't have so much power over me.

One thing I found interesting in your book was about 'breaking up properly' with a friend, which can be a necessary (yet scary) thing. How have you dealt with a friendship break-up in the past without getting clammy-handed and anxiety-fuelled?

Oh God. Since I wrote the book, I've broken up with a friend. It was this girl I used to live with and when I moved out, I thought our friendship was over because we fought a bit. She obviously didn't and kept asking me for coffee and catch-ups. I just texted her one day and said I wasn't comfortable continuing the friendship, and I wished her well but didn't want to be in her life any more. I nearly threw up, it felt so unnatural and weird to be so honest. We are trained, especially as women, to be likeable and polite. My people pleasing instinct was strong but my feeling that she shouldn't be in my life was stronger. I could've tried being vague or I could have ghosted her but it didn't feel right. Ultimately, I think it was a kindness to tell her rather than leave her guessing or be rude to her. I feel OK about it now, but it was a confronting thing to do. I'd say it's perfectly fine to craft a thoughtful, clear text message to break up with someone, and it's definitely preferable to just disappearing and leaving them to wonder what they did wrong. Every friendship is different so I'd really encourage people to end them in whatever way feels right.

You've written agony aunt-style friendship advice columns for hugely popular publications – do you have any tips for tackling toxic friendships? I bet you're asked this a lot!

Such a good question! If you've got a toxic friend, it helps to identify it. Red flags include:

- People who shower you with affection and generosity only to withdraw from you.
- People who criticise you or put you down.
- People who try to isolate you from your other friends.
- If someone is hurting you, undermining your confidence, trying to turn you against people you love or trying to control you, it's important that you extricate yourself safely from that friendship.

We're getting better at recognising the signs of a toxic romantic relationship, but we need to be vigilant with friendships too.

What's one of the most important lessons you've learnt from writing *The Friendship Cure*?

That loneliness does not discriminate! That any one of us can get lonely, no matter how old or how successful or even how popular. That it's possible to be lonely even when you're in a crowded room of people. That actively cultivating and protecting your friends is one of the smartest things you can do for your mental and physical health.

Finally, from making new friends to being your own best friend, do you have any words of wisdom or mantras that members of The Insecure Girls' Club can add to their repertoire?

Friendship is, ideally, an exchange of vulnerabilities. Vulnerability is the quickest shortcut to intimacy. Virtually everyone gets lonely so don't chastise yourself for it.

COMMUNICATION, COMMUNICATION, COMMUNICATION

If ever there was a situation at school involving upset or tears after some typical bitchiness, my dad always insisted that talking it out and communicating properly was the best thing to do. He'd get frustrated when I'd say, 'No! I'll just text her!' and always argued a phone call would be the best solution. I hate to say it, but he was right (even though the thought of a phone call to resolve a fallout still gives me nervous butterflies). Texts can be misconstrued and often things can get taken out of context. If you think the scales of a friendship are off balance, communication is the key to keeping everyone's expectations in check. If someone is expecting to catch up with you and you've been snowed under, let them know. Try to avoid leaving it to the very last minute to cancel plans; if you don't think you'll be able to make it to an event, the earlier you say so the better. If you've laid things out clearly for someone to see, it's not up to you how they perceive it.

My friend Lucy once said, 'Hold up a mirror before you hold up a magnifying glass,'[30] and if you're feeling ready to criticise a pal for dropping the ball, I think this is a perfect reminder that not everyone is perfect. Check your own habits before you criticise friends. If you're feeling lonely because someone hasn't texted you, consider if you've texted them and checked in recently. If not, text them to meet up; don't wait for them to do it. Try not to treat friendship like a game, and instead remember that communication is king and friendship is a two-way street.

One invaluable friend told me she tries to view text messages and WhatsApps like letters (obviously providing it's not a matter of high urgency or *'Where are you, I've been waiting half an hour?!'*). If it's a long message, she said you should be able to take time over it. Letters never arrived in five minutes, so give yourself a break and take care when you need to.

PLEASE YOURSELF BEFORE OTHERS

Learning to set boundaries and be assertive can be scary, but it shows that you respect and value yourself, which is a pretty cool thing indeed.

Here are some of my favourite tips for learning to stand your own ground in a polite and manageable way: no nerves needed!
- Give yourself a little pat on the back if you manage to say no when you'd normally say yes. Don't overthink it once it's been said, but feel relief that you considered your own needs and reward yourself by not questioning whether you did the right thing.

- Suggest an alternative. If you need to let someone down, suggest an alternative to ease the guilt you might feel. 'I love seeing you but I really need to get on with this project this week. How about we do something in a couple of weeks instead?'
- Begin small. If you have a preference in a situation, voice it. If your friend suggests going to see a horror film at the cinema, there's no problem saying you'd rather see something else instead. Try to make your voice heard in situations where you'd otherwise be indifferent, and practise letting people know what you'd rather do.
- Know your limits. Just because you're friends with someone doesn't mean you have to share everything with them. You don't have to be available all the time and they don't have to know the intricacies of your life either. That doesn't make the friendship less important, but don't feel obliged to tell people everything if you'd rather not.

And finally, what's the worst that can happen? Your friends should respect your own time and wellbeing as much as their own. You deserve to be listened to, so start small and practise flexin' that muscle of pleasing yourself first.

KNOW THAT YOU CAN'T WIN 'EM ALL

In a world with so many voices, personalities, tastes, quirks, backgrounds and interests, your special unique quality is simply being you. Don't try and water yourself down to make everyone like you. Instead, embrace everything about yourself wholly – your loud laugh, curiosity, knack for remembering random facts but never birthdays, terrible taste in party songs but amazing dance moves, appalling dad jokes and nervousness to try new things. All of these things make up one brilliant individual who doesn't need to make everyone happy – because that's a pressure none of us needs. The same goes for friends – a friend might not be able to be everything to you, but appreciate the things they are instead of what they aren't.

If you ever struggle to think of the things that make you so brilliant, here are a few ideas:
- List five things you like about yourself. This sounds simple, but sometimes it can be tricky. If you struggle, ask someone who knows you and you trust – I'm sure they'd be more than happy to point out all your best bits.
- Look at your past experiences. Perhaps you've been there for a friend during a difficult time, helped a pal with a personal project, or stayed

late at work when a colleague needed the support. These are all brilliant qualities you maybe didn't even realise you had. Is there anything else you're proud of? Write. It. Down!

- Although to some they might sound cheesy, get yourself some of the affirmation cards I mentioned before. Written in the first person, affirmation cards are there with positive reminders and confidence-boosting statements for when you need some reassurance (for example, 'I am capable', 'I am trying my best'). Having them handy for a one-to-one pep talk can be the little pick-me-up you need.

- Forgive and forget! If you're someone who continually guilt trips and shames yourself for past experiences, try to forgive yourself and remind yourself that those things don't have to shape you. Don't let past mistakes govern the way you view yourself. We are constantly changing and evolving, so let go of past judgement errors and wrongdoing. Nobody is perfect – and we are not the product of every mistake we've made.

Takeaway pick-me-ups for forging friendships and being the best mate you can be, from The Insecure Girls' Club

- With friendships, remember – quality over quantity. Focus on the friends you have, and water them like a bunch of your favourite peonies (they'll seriously droop otherwise).
- When making new friends, follow your interests. Whether it's learning a new skill, joining a club, going to a shopping event or a live podcast, if you follow your interests you'll always have a common ground.
- Know that having no friendship at all is better than having one that makes you feel bad about yourself. Not every friendship will last forever, and if you can take a lesson from it then it'll never be a total waste of your time.
- If you find it hard to switch off, or you feel too available, turn off 'read' receipts and notifications. You don't have to see those little WhatsApp ticks turn blue and feel like you're constantly on a countdown to reply.
- Hold up a mirror before you hold up a magnifying glass. Always.
- Remember that sometimes people pleasing is a good thing, but more often than not it's a sign to start thinking about your own needs. Start small with assertiveness and build up to feeling more confident in creating your own boundaries.

- The most important opinion is the one you have of yourself. You can't change the way other people think about you, but you can change the way you think of yourself. Use daily reminders to pick yourself up when needed.

6

'But are my ideas good enough?': stepping stones to self-belief

Being your own PR gal/cheerleader is the best way of getting there

Without any prior experience in PR, when I started my blog nearly ten years ago I initially found it nigh on impossible to champion myself and my ideas. Not that you need a degree in PR or marketing to have a little faith in yourself, but I truly believed I'd have more success trying to promote a chocolate teapot than I would anything I'd done on my own. Each time I shared a Facebook update with a link to a new blog post, I'd silently worry that people would have a snort-fuelled chuckle about it with each other.

When it came to putting together a book proposal, one of the hardest things to say in meetings was, 'Hey! There's a real gap in the market for this book, and I'm the person to do this work.' Even though I *knew* there was a place in the market and I'd *tried* my absolute best, my internal voice was saying, 'Mm, well I'm sure it'll be *all right* – hopefully it won't be shit. Oh God, it might be a bit shit. Oh, never mind.'

And often, that's exactly what halts self-belief in its tracks. We downplay our successes, undermine our achievements, listen to our noisy inner critic, and let others dive into their opinions on our ideas before we've even had a chance to believe in them ourselves. Suddenly every negative comment or mistake we've made in the past frames our present experiences. No matter what kind of industry you work in – creative, corporate or otherwise – having faith in your ability and ideas is the key to growth; but how do we actually do it?

You've made it this far, so you'll know how crucial self-belief is. Doubting ourselves is a self-defeating cycle that will ultimately stop us doing the things we want to do. I've learnt, very gradually, that self-belief isn't something that comes overnight, but it is something that can be practised. It's a work in progress, and much like building a house it requires solid foundations. Nobody starts off being perfect at anything, and even the most successful people have to rehearse before getting it right. Look at Emma Stone's character Mia in the film *La La Land*! How many bad auditions did she endure before she finally hit the big time as an actress? Lots. If it hadn't have been for her self-belief, she'd have packed it in when nobody showed up at her disastrous play opening, and stopped learning lines after hearing some dismissive feedback. But our girl E.S. carried on, picked herself up and made it! Life doesn't always turn out like a feel-good film, but if we give up on our dreams, the world simply carries on, and we'll inevitably miss out.

So, pick up your pom-poms, dust off your eighties

motivational playlist, and perhaps re-watch *La La Land* to crystallise that last reference. We have some believin' to do . . .

BELIEVING IN YOURSELF
BEFORE OTHERS DO

When a friend who inspires you is feeling negative about herself, you wonder how on earth she could feel that way when she has so much going for her – why can she not see it?! But do you apply the same logic when you're feeling negative yourself? Often, believing in ourselves is a hundred times more challenging than giving it out. We can see possibility so clearly in others, but sometimes recognising it in ourselves is trickier.

And the reason it's so important we're cheerleading for ourselves? Because you can't always rely on others to do the cheering for you. Take a recent experience I had with a friend. I'd been sharing my problems with her over lunch, worrying work hadn't been going quite as well as I'd hoped and feeling a bit lacklustre. Rather than telling me I was doing OK (which, although perhaps a bit self-indulgent, was absolutely what I was after), she began sharing how she was feeling rubbish at work too. Even though this was *absolutely fair enough*, I realised I'd been relying on her to pick me up, and when I didn't get that from her I felt even worse. She was absolutely within her rights not to big me up if I was subconsciously fishing for a bit of a boost, and it made me realise that we can't always rely on others to do the work for us – because honestly? If we're constantly seeking validation from others we might never get the assurance we need to truly realise how brilliant we are. We end up pinning all of our belief on what we hope other people will say about us, when really we need to achieve it for ourselves.

. . . .

'I'd tell myself not to place my value in other people. I thought too much of what other people thought, and allowed myself to be treated badly because I didn't know my own value. It was a hard lesson to learn, but a necessary one.'

GHENET, *London*

. . . .

IS THIS EVEN ANY GOOD?

When an idea first enters the world, it's rarely a fully formed thing. It could be a twinkle in your eye, or a little golden thread ready to be pulled to unravel something brilliant. You might need to run for your nearest notebook or pull up your iPhone notes before it vanishes – but whatever it is, having confidence in it, talking about it and building on it will make it stronger.

Growing up, I had endless ideas for magazines I would one day publish, fashion shows I'd design for, stage and model in (ten-year-old me had an enviable amount of confidence), plays I'd write that would become films, and career paths that would require everything from veterinary science degrees to extensive ice skating training. From all those ideas, I was able to get a real sense of self and discover the things that truly lit me up and sparked my passion. Having belief in your own ideas, however ill formed or out-there, makes them better; and if you believe in them, other people are likely to do so too.

DON'T DO YOURSELF A DISSERVICE

Although 'fake it till you make it' isn't the coolest phrase to have pinned to your inspiration board, having conviction when talking about something – whether you're asking for a pay rise or putting yourself forward for a role – means you'll almost certainly be met with a positive response. Typically, my natural instinct is to apologise before I've even started, approach a new possibility with scepticism and tell others I don't deserve it – but going in confident (even if you're feeling wobbly) is the key to having other people believe in what you're saying.

Thinking that you don't deserve to be doing something or to be at that table is sometimes down to the insecurity that follows us when new experiences come knocking. It's years of imposter syndrome, feeling like there isn't space for us, and an unfamiliar moment all bundled up into one. This is the time when we need a bit of self-belief the most, yet often it's when self-belief is the hardest thing to find.

In these moments, keeping your insecurity to yourself and voicing it afterwards is sometimes best. I've been at glamorous events where I've said to the host, 'I don't know why I'm here,' in a moment of unfiltered insecurity – but to them, this could be a minor alarm bell that they've made a mistake and invited the wrong person. Similarly, don't tell your managing director that you feel like you're about to be 'sussed out' and that it's a fluke you're even in the meeting. The last thing you want is them worrying they've offered you too much money or too many responsibilities. Try to remember that they've chosen you to be there for a reason, and (unless you literally weren't invited and sneaked in!) you can sit back and give yourself an enormous pat on the back for getting into that room – because you deserve to be there. Don't do yourself a disservice by making anyone else think otherwise.

Deeba Syed
political activist and sexual harassment lawyer

I am in awe of the work Deeba (@deebaalinasyed) is doing across politics and law for women's rights – she helped launch Rights of Women, the only free helpline for women in England and Wales who have been sexually harassed at work. Both areas can feel like a minefield to navigate as a woman, and talking to Deeba I couldn't be more inspired by her vision and determination. From set-backs and detaching from criticism to oozing the confidence of a mediocre man, we discussed self-belief and how to carry on when the going gets tough . . .

Deeba, you tirelessly campaign for women's rights – how did you find your way into law and activism?
I've been an activist for nearly nine years now. I honestly never imagined when I was younger that I would be so involved in activism or politics. I never felt very powerful and always assumed I couldn't have much impact in the world. I have no connections or anything like that. I never studied politics and to be honest I always assumed that was for boys. But I just wanted to throw myself in. I thought the best way I could learn

about it was to work for an MP, so I wrote this really long and cringe email to every shadow cabinet member at the time, saying I didn't know much about politics but that I would work very hard and to please give me a shot.

To my utter surprise, one MP actually got back to me. I worked for free at first, managing this MP's diary and working in a bar in the evenings, but it became apparent to me that no matter what I did, I could never earn people's respect on an intellectual level. Men were always deemed to be the default of where to go to for policy and political advice; women were only ever consulted for advice on how to run events, photo shoots, aesthetics. Never strategy. Never decision making. It made me feel so angry. I would think, hey – I'm smarter than this.

When I began following you, one of my favourite posts of yours was seeing you talk about proving people wrong when it came to feeling unconfident at school and moving into law with dyslexia. How did you overcome the negative voices that told you that you couldn't?
Yes, I'm very dyslexic. It took me ages to learn how to read when I was a kid. I was held back at school because I couldn't say the alphabet properly. It made me very self-conscious growing up; I suppose when you struggle like that you have a distorted image of your value. I would struggle to do things that I saw other people around me do so easily. I thought it meant I wasn't clever, which meant I didn't have as much to offer. I ended up rebelling against it all and decided I wasn't going to be academic. I didn't believe dyslexia was a 'gift' like people say; I thought it was a curse that meant I would never succeed, so I thought, why bother?

I think dyslexics are quite used to getting things wrong,

feeling a bit embarrassed and not excelling easily. I think it makes us tougher. More resilient. We are really good at taking knocks, dusting ourselves off and getting back up again, because we are more used to it. I think my dyslexia has given me drive, real determination to succeed, because naturally the hurdles have always been that bit higher for me. But that determination can count for a lot, sometimes more than natural ability. I wanted to push myself, really hard, to prove to myself that I could do it, and to make up for that lost time when I didn't believe in myself.

So much of what feeds into day-to-day insecurity is the inability to trust our own judgement. When it comes to politics and having our own opinion online, how can we push our insecurities to one side and hush our inner critic that says, 'You don't know enough about this!'?
To be honest, I still struggle with this all the time. It's taken me so long to believe in myself! Sometimes I just remind myself to have all the confidence of a mediocre white man. I thought this a lot when I worked in Parliament; I would hear political advisers speak up in meetings and command such gravitas and respect. I would think, 'I was just thinking that, why didn't I say it?'. It takes practice; the more you do it, the easier it becomes.

What are your biggest tips for silencing your inner critic? Do you ever have moments when you doubt your ability, and how do you overcome those?
Of course I do! Public speaking makes me dizzy with anxiety sometimes. When I first started doing it, I once got it so bad I actually wanted to run off the stage and vomit. But the more

I've done it, the easier it has become. I've been able to do TV and radio, which I could never have dreamed of a few years ago. Set yourself small challenges and succeed at them; then you can look back at all the baby steps and see how far they can really go, added up.

I find it useful to have a chat with someone who's knowledgeable about the subject too. I hate email (a dyslexic's nightmare); I much prefer to talk on the phone. And I don't mind asking dumb questions. I will literally ask anything, even if it might sound stupid. You have to ask for help, and you just have to admit when you don't understand something. So, when that voice tells you to shut up and not look stupid, just go ahead and speak up instead.

What has been the biggest lesson you've learnt from your experience campaigning, and what would you say to sixteen-year-old Deeba?
Sixteen-year-old Deeba would think I'm so uncool! Now I spend my Saturdays at political conferences or on marches. Then all I cared about was boys and Lou Reed. I honestly don't think I would even have been able to tell you who was prime minister. I've changed a lot. All the little trials and tribulations have changed me. I've seen everything I've been through and survived it all. I tell myself I can do anything now, and it's been the most important thing I could have ever learnt.

I take huge inspiration from outspoken sisters who have come before me. I love how fearless and gobby people like Jess Phillips MP are; she isn't afraid of anything. Sometimes when I'm not sure if I should post or tweet something, I think, 'Would Jess?' And if I think yes, that tends to be a good thing.

I also really look up to activists like Malala Yousafzai and

200

Emma Watson, who have different styles but are both so intelligent and articulate. They deliver such powerful messages of hope with such dignity and grace. I prefer activism to be positive like this.

Finally, you're a woman with lots of invaluable experience. Do you have any words of compassion or mantras that members of The Insecure Girls' Club can add to their repertoire?

I feel like I've been through a few battles and have the scars to show it, especially being involved in politics. I think activism is wonderful, but political activism can be vicious. I've had ups and downs with it. You have to remember why you're doing it and always be able to go back to that reason when things get hard. So, my mantra is to remember your 'why'. You have to be thick-skinned in politics; change is never easy and if you came to be liked, you came to the wrong place! We all have to decide what we think is right and fight for that.

IT'S THE CLIMB!

One of the keys to having faith in yourself is to start small. If you're constantly looking at enormous goals and not quite reaching them, you're going to struggle to tick off the bigger things. My sister-in-law Lucy always reminds me of the funny yet brilliant saying, 'When eating an elephant, take one bite at a time' (from US Army General Creighton Abrams) – if you're faced with something big, breaking it down into small bites is the best way to get it done. Whether that's your savings goal, career steps or feeling better about yourself, take small steps – removing negative body talk one day at a time, saving £20 a week, or signing up for a night course in that new hobby you want to try.

Similarly, my friend Charlotte taught me that, 'If you never try it or put it out there, you can never improve on it'. It was a throwaway comment, but it's affected my work ethic enormously. Sometimes our acceptance that we're just not 'good' at something stops us at the first hurdle. You'll never hit the peak of a mountain unless you begin at the bottom, and you'll never feel confident in that rainbow-sequinned party dress until you give it a whirl. We are so quick to build our own glass ceiling that we forget smashing it could be a possibility.

Appreciating the journey along the way can be one of the biggest pleasures of success – especially if we realise that there is never really a peak. In *How to Be a Grown-Up*, Daisy Buchanan writes: 'If you're creative, or ambitious, or a bit of a perfectionist, you'll never reach the top and the journey will never make you happy unless you learn to appreciate the climb itself.'[31] Embracing the journey (or 'The Climb', as the wise Miley Cyrus once said) can be the real definition of success.

TRUST YOUR GUT

Do you feel confident in trusting your gut?

Yes: 65% | No: 25% | Don't know: 10%

You know that knee-jerk reaction you have to something you're *so* sure about? For me it usually comes when asked which film I want to watch on a Sunday evening (*'Pretty Woman!'*), or it's an intuitive reaction to a big work commitment ('I know that project isn't for me,' or 'Yes, I'll be there with bells on.'). But it could be any number of things – whether a new job is right for you or an old relationship is worth sticking at or even a bigger decision, which might require catching a few Zs before you cement it for good. It's only in the last few years that I have really learnt how powerful it is to listen to my gut.

Often we know the answer to a big question from the beginning, but because we have so little belief in our own opinions, we seek validation first – even if it's not the validation we need. Your gut reaction is your body or mind subtly giving you signs and telling you exactly what you think is right, so when it comes to believing in yourself, you're the person that has it spot on. This feeling can often be mistaken for fear or anxiety bubbling away in the pit of your stomach, and it doesn't mean you need to make a rash decision, but treat it as a protective agent, looking out for you when you need it most. It feels daunting at first (listening to yourself over the words of others is a skill that takes practice), but it's something you can definitely start tuning in to and trusting over time.

KNOW THAT MISTAKES
AREN'T PERMANENT

In life, not everything will go to plan. You might not get the grades you want, you might end up not getting into your chosen university, you might say something in the heat of the moment that you go on to regret, and you might not get the job you've had your heart set on the first time you apply. Try not to put too much value on those moments. Don't hold on to guilt for every silly thing you've said, and don't dwell on your wrongdoings if you know you want to change and be better. Going wrong isn't the end of the road. You can look back on your mistakes to drive you forwards, but don't let them frame everything you go on to do.

**What do you say to remind yourself
that things will be OK?**

'It's fine – you have done this before. (Normally it is something that I have done a million times and I just need to
remind myself I'm OK.)'   *Amey, Aberdeen*

Sometimes, things going wrong pave the way for something going right – and even far better. Look at Elizabeth
Day's *How To Fail* podcast. Her guests are some of the
most remarkable women in the world (including Dame
Kelly Holmes and Gina Miller) – all discussing the things
that went wrong, which have led them to where they are
now. There are times when I didn't get a job I wanted, when
I was looking for a place to live but flats came and went,
when relationships with past boyfriends didn't go to plan.
But if those things hadn't happened, would I be where I am
now? It's unlikely.

*Try to see your mistakes as 'experience tokens' that
you can cash in for the feeling, 'I overcame that!'*

LET'S RECAP!

....

We've tackled the importance of being your own biggest cheerleader (who really needs the Wildcats?), stepping away from external validation, fakin' it till we make it, aiming to have enough self-belief that we don't feel compelled to tell the big cheese we should be looking at redundancy instead of a promotion, and realising that our mistakes aren't everything. Navigating self-belief is a tricky process – but we're getting there, gang!

STOP RIGHT NOW,
THANK YOU VERY MUCH

So, how can we put all this into practice? How can we look after ourselves day-to-day so that we feel armed and ready when we're struck with a wobble? Can we find a way to appreciate how far we've come, and can we measure what it is that's so important to us in the first place?

BEING YOUR OWN CHEERLEADER

If, like me, you find yourself waiting for other people to cheer you on, then turn things around. I've learnt that I can't always rely on someone else to make me feel better about myself and I need to do that work myself. Ironically, sometimes a push in the wrong direction from someone else makes you realise that wasn't where you wanted to be going. I've become a lot better at taking stock of the great things I have going on in my career and giving myself a little one-on-one appraisal. I look at the things that are making me feel 'less than' and start thinking of what I'd say to a friend in my position. For example:

- 'I'm sorry things aren't great at the moment – but look what you were up to last month/week/year! These things always have ebbs and flows, and you've done some amazing things this year.'
- 'You're so creative – why don't you harness that in the meantime and work on the projects you've been putting to one side?'
- 'Don't see it as a defeat – see it as a challenge that you'll overcome.'

It might sound as cheesy as giving yourself a TEDx talk in the mirror, but you'd be surprised at how much difference it makes when you detach from that external validation and start recognising your achievements, no matter how big or small, for yourself.

Write down all of your strengths, or simply scroll through your own Instagram feed to pick out some of the things you've felt proud of in the last year. They don't have to be momentous, but every article you've pitched, exam you've taken or charity run you've blitzed is worth adding to a mental 'did-do' list, which you can remember as 'can do' things that you are more than capable of. Give me a 'YOU'! Give me a 'GOT'! Give me a 'THIS'!

STOP DOWNPLAYING YOUR SUCCESSES

When this book was first commissioned, I found it so hard to believe I was actually being asked to write a real-life, available-in-Waterstones book that I downplayed it so much that some of my family and friends didn't actually think I was writing a '*book* book'. It was my own fault. My muted reaction to it (prompted by my desire not to come off as 'braggy') guided the reactions of others, so despite the fact that writing a book had been a huge goal for me, the news was met with whelm (neither overwhelm nor underwhelm, FYI): not what I'd been expecting.

May this be a lesson for anyone who's just ticked off a huge achievement – shout about it! Send a bell crier into the centre of town on market day (lol) and let the world know that *you've done it*. As I said before, you can't wait for other people to validate your own feelings and successes, so let people know when they happen. By making people aware of one thing going right, you're opening yourself up for other great things to happen (for example, if you let your manager know a thrilled customer sent you a letter to thank you for your service, she's far more likely to promote you, or at least give you the pat on the back you've earned). It's good, girl – so celebrate it!

'But are my ideas good enough?'

. . . .

'On some days I have to consciously interrupt my stream of negative thoughts to remind myself of all the great, or even mediocre, things I've recently accomplished. It's about being able to be your own biggest support when you most need it, and having the ability to say, "But look at all the qualities I do have."'

SAADIYA, *London*

. . . .

TREAT SITUATIONS AS IF THEY WEREN'T YOUR OWN

What is the best piece of advice someone has given you?

'Never measure yourself using someone else's ruler.'
Becky, London

When things start going wrong and you're met with a fork in the road, deal with it as if you were talking to a friend. You wouldn't tell them to just give up and pack it all in; you'd give them alternative solutions or ways to overcome the failure. If you don't get the job you applied for, rather than telling yourself how rubbish you are, think what you'd tell a friend who got a rejection: 'Something better will come along – things are always working out', 'It's their loss – they didn't deserve you anyway!'. If you'd say it to a friend in all honesty, then say it to yourself too. Every time you offer a friend great advice or give them a stellar pick-me-up, write it down somewhere safe and pull it out for when you need it too – if it's good enough for the people you love the most, it's absolutely good enough for you.

What we say *vs* what we should say

Who invited me here?! I honestly have no idea why I'm at this.
It's so exciting to be here! It's so nice to be included and invited to something like this.

Um, it'd be nice to talk about maybe seeing if there's any scope for slightly more responsibility in this role – only if that's OK?
I'd love to chat about my role, and the potential for more responsibility. I've worked really hard lately, and it'd be great to chat about things!

Oh, so I'm doing this thing, it's not anything that exciting. But yeah.
I'm doing X, I can't believe it! I've worked so hard, and it's so surreal, but YES!

I didn't get the job – I knew I wouldn't, ugh.
I'm sure something better will crop up. One thing falls apart so something else can fall together, isn't that what they say? It's their loss!

DO SOME PERSONAL MEASURING

It's easy to be under the illusion that you need to conform to certain social benchmarks to think you're doing well. If you're not feeling great about your achievements or yourself, seeing endless marriage proposals, new houses, job promotions and growing follower counts can lead us to believe that we should be ticking these things off too, and that these are the things we want to accomplish ourselves. But do we even want them for ourselves or are we just socially conditioned to want them? Sometimes we can make ourselves believe these things will make us feel secure and happy, but if we achieve them and they don't, we're at a loss.

THE INSECURE GIRL'S HANDBOOK

What would your dream five-year plan look like? Step away from Instagram and the pile of *Town & Country* magazines in your mum's house – what does success look like for *you*?

- Does the idea of starting a family fill you with joy – or are you ready to pack your bags and head across the world for some *Eat Pray Love* action? Map out three–five things that you'd love to one day achieve and let them be the light that guides you to your goals. They can be as small or significant as you like, personal or career-related. Perhaps you'd love to train for a marathon, finally get that tattoo, or jump into a new career. Maybe it's buying your own home – figure out what your ideal scenario looks like, work backwards to where you are, then decide what needs to be done to get there.

- Start with the next six months, then build up to a year, and then onwards. Do you want to save for a flat deposit, for example? Start with a small amount week on week, or month on month, and build up a little more if you find it's achievable. If you know you can afford to be putting aside more of your monthly pay packet, then start a savings account for it.

- Remember, five years is only a starting point. If things take longer, that's not a sign of defeat. Setting a time limit for your goals is a way of kick-starting them and driving you forward, and shouldn't apply unwanted pressure (there's enough of that as it is)! Take your time, and know that if you need longer to reach your goal it won't make it any less worthwhile.

Whatever your goal, take each day as it comes. It's far easier to implement steps to what you want when you know what they are – but taking them one at a time is the key to not getting overwhelmed. Your plan is there to help you focus on what you want, not something to stress yourself out with. It's as flexible as you are – and you are in charge of your own goalposts. If something doesn't happen in the timeframe you'd like, make the goalposts a little wider. No harm done.

Also remember that we can forget our own tastes and desires when presented with other people's. I know that when I'm sitting at home, I can become swept up in others' holiday photos – be it blue skies in Bali, breathtaking sunsets in Mumbai or zip-wiring in New Zealand; far-flung destinations which, until that moment, I'd perhaps never had any true desire to visit. A bit of time out can remind me that really, my idea of heaven is the British seaside – but it's so easy to forget that when you're focusing on other people's ideals of happiness. However, if looking at someone's holiday photos gives you a pang of envy, or makes you feel 'less than', question why. Is it because that place is somewhere you've always dreamt of heading to, or are you feeling crappy about work at the moment and looking for any sort of escape? We must name and claim our insecurities because they will lead us to what it is we truly want – and therein lies our ability to motivate ourselves to work hard for what it is we really want to achieve. Magic, right?

LOOK AFTER YOURSELF

One of my favourite Dolly Alderton quotes came from a piece she wrote for the brilliant book *Life Honestly*. She says: 'If you take in big thoughts and clever voices, you'll cultivate big thoughts and a clever voice.'[32] A big part of fostering self-belief and feeling capable is showing yourself some TLC and putting in a bit of work to help you along the way.

You could:
- Read more novels on the train to work if you want to become a better reader (or, like me, start using bigger words) – library cards are the key here!
- Listen to a variety of podcasts if you want to have broader conversations (I remember when

my mum started listening to LBC on her way to work and then became *very* topical all of a sudden).

- Start going to ballet classes or salsa with a friend after work if you want to become better at dancing (or just whip on a playlist as you clean the kitchen, and start wrigglin' those hips).
- Try practising yoga (at home or a studio) if you want to feel stronger. You don't need to have the best gear or be the most flexible to gently start moving your body.
- Pick up some watercolours from an art store if you want to become better at painting.
- Make your favourite dishes for dinner from scratch, and play around with new ones (try using up every leftover in your fridge) if you want to get better at cooking – and also nourish yourself at the same time, bonus!

You get the gist. To have more belief in yourself, you have to start flexing the muscle of the thing you want to get better at – remember, it's never too late to start.

. . . .

'I am enough in this moment, but also there is always something small I can do today that will help my tomorrow.'

SARAH, *Chichester*

. . . .

Saima Thompson

restaurateur, Trekstock ambassador and writer

Having begun her multi-award-winning restaurant Masala Wala Cafe in 2015 with her mum and their home-cooked recipes, Saima knows a thing or two about trusting your instincts and championing self-belief. Additionally, with her stage-four cancer diagnosis, Saima has proved to be a beacon of light on and offline, starting a BAME cancer support group and sharing her story openly. From being authentic to following your gut, this lady is a wise one indeed . . .

Saima, you're a writer, you speak honestly about your experience with cancer, and you're a kick-ass restaurateur. How did that all begin – how did you turn that idea into a reality? I opened the restaurant back in 2015 with my mum, and I could give some elaborate love story about how the cuisine needs to be spread up and down the country – but the truth is that I simply tried to convince my mum to open a restaurant and she said yes. She was a Punjabi homemaker, an immigrant mother who came over in the eighties, had four children, had never worked, and had to create an employment opportunity for both of us that would work. Every Pakistani homemaker makes incredible food at home, and I don't think that this is shared enough. These recipes are passed down from generation to generation but they all just stay inside the family kitchens, so I thought, 'Why not share it around the restaurant scene?' And from day one it was well received.

Starting a business is a scary step for anyone. How did you become your own biggest cheerleader?
Ultimately, I believed in the product, I believed in the recipes, and I just thought that the food would speak for itself. We were cooking the food during the day and serving at night for the first six months when we opened, and for me to learn and spend that time with my mum was really precious – not a lot of people have the opportunity to spend such an intense time with their parents. You spend all of your teenage years trying to get away from your parents through embarrassment – even for me, my thoughts growing up were that I didn't want to smell like curry and I would close the kitchen door. So now it's quite funny that in my adult years I've kind of embraced my roots, and I suppose that came through a desire for authenticity. I wanted to understand who I was, being a British Pakistani, and that's where the confidence came with the business; it felt like coming home.

Did you have to learn to trust your gut?
I'd say yes. I think that your gut is your second brain, and you have to go with your gut instincts. The one thing that I would say is that I probably didn't do enough research. I did go with my gut a lot, and a lot of the time it paid off. In the build-up to opening, I could have had a bit more self-belief – so there were a lot of conflicting feelings and a lot of nervousness. But

218

I think that's the case with anything – when you're taking a risk there's always a lot of self-doubt and imposter syndrome. Going from someone who worked in retail management to a self-employed managing restaurateur is a big leap and I had to fight those demons, but the trust and the offering was there. I think we're still the only mother/daughter Pakistani restaurant offering in the UK.

After being diagnosed with stage-four lung cancer, you have been such a ray of light to so many – sharing your story, speaking publicly and setting up a BAME support group on top of running Masala Wala Cafe. What's been the most important thing you've learnt?
What I wanted to get out of speaking publicly about it was to reach out to other people of colour. What I found was that, in this day and age, being a young person with cancer is quite isolating at the best of times, but being someone of colour, I saw a lot of white women sharing their stories, but didn't see much of me – and the best thing about the internet is that it's never been easier to find your own tribe, or even create your own tribe. I hope that through me sharing my story, somebody else who might get diagnosed won't feel so alone. In the early days (of diagnosis), I felt so isolated at times, and I suffered from post-traumatic stress which I do talk openly about, because again it is another side of cancer, the mental side, that I don't think gets talked about enough. There's a lot of, 'You can fight this,' 'You've got this, girl,' but doctors have come a long way to be able to treat it; it's them fighting it, not me! A lot of it is the mental battle – you have to go home and live with it and adapt your life around it, and look to live purposefully with it. Even friends have done the sideways sympa-

thetic head tilt followed by, 'So what are the doctors saying?'. But I'm so much more than that. I've had such a fulfilling life before the diagnosis; I have to carry this with me now. That's the beauty of reaching out online, and trying to find people who things hadn't gone the right way for. I was looking for resilient stories. I think we're sold this idea that you grow up to be just one thing and that's it. But it can be multi-faceted. So I can be a cancer patient, a restaurateur, a daughter, a wife; I can be all these things. I've got to carry this diagnosis with me: I'm not just a poor cancer patient.

It's a serious skill to master, but what are your top tips for garnering self-belief?
I think firstly, taking time. Secondly, loving yourself and people around you. I've learnt that now. It sounds so cheesy, but just making sure that you check in with yourself, and love yourself, and have gratitude as well. It's going back to basics, such simple things. Before the diagnosis, I thought that everything about me was in my head, and now I appreciate my body, and how it can regenerate itself and do all of these wonderful things. It's recovering and going through cancer – I'm just a bit more grateful now. Having your health is important, having a roof over your head is important; if you have those things then you're smashing it!

Finally, you're a woman with lots of brilliant wisdom – do you have any words of compassion or mantras that members of The Insecure Girls' Club can add to their repertoire?
You do not have to be anything or anyone, you are perfect just the way you are, and can damn well do what you want, when you want.

YOU'VE DONE THIS ALREADY!

It can take a number of things going right to make you realise you've done this all before. Look over your CV, or make one if you haven't got one already. I did this a few years ago when, after being self-employed for a few years and shrouded in doubt, I began to wonder if I was even employable! I downloaded a CV template, popped down my achievements as if I was applying for a job, and listed the exams, skills and projects I was proud of, which gave me a subtle reminder that perhaps I was more qualified than I believed. It's so easy to forget how much you've done already and fail to celebrate all the transferrable skills you've collected.

Write your own alternative CV:
- Download a CV template (if in doubt, Etsy has some great ones), and think back on all of the things you've done.
- Maybe you've just finished some exams (which means, whatever the results, you are driven and willing to learn) or perhaps you've just started a Saturday job. List those education and career-related achievements.
- Also look at your extra-curricular pursuits. Do you write a blog? This shows you have a passion

for a certain topic and perhaps even a knack for coding, writing and photography. Have you performed in a local production, or do you have a love for illustrating on the side?

- Then there are the things you probably don't even realise you're doing. For example, have you helped a friend run an event or taken part in a charity bake sale? All of these things show responsibility, organisation, initiative and more, plus they add colour to your CV.

Take all of these things as small signs that you are capable, and use them in your 'pick-me-up' arsenal for when you're not feeling so great.

AND, BABES! WHAT IF IT ALL GOES RIGHT?

You've made it this far in life, and you're here! You're breathing – and you're you! You've made enough good decisions to get you to this very day, and what if all this hard work *does* pay off? Often we view each decision with a fatalistic perspective: 'Oh God, what if this all goes terribly wrong?', 'What if I've said the wrong thing *again*?', 'Why would that happen for me?'. But clearly your judgement isn't so bad (you did pick up this book, after all). For every time you think, 'This is going to go terribly wrong,' try flipping it on its head: 'What if this goes brilliantly right?'. If we're brave enough to give something a try, then surely we can be brave enough to assume the best-case scenario too. Self-belief won't always change the outcome in life, and manifesting 'good vibes' doesn't mean things always go swimmingly, but if we believe we're doing the best we can do for ourselves, that's really all that matters.

. . . .

'I like to remind myself about the possibility of things that lie ahead. I'm facing up to depression at the moment, after keeping it buried away for years. It's become even more important to be kind to myself and to tell myself everything will be OK. I love the part in Matt Haig's *Reasons to Stay Alive* where he talks about all the things that have yet to happen in your life that will make you feel joy. It comforts me so much and it's something I read over and over again. For me it's books I've yet to read, conversations I haven't yet had, dogs I haven't patted, gigs I haven't been to, cities I've yet to hold my boyfriend's hand in.'

SARAH, *London*

. . . .

Takeaway pick-me-ups to keep on believin', from The Insecure Girls' Club

- If you have an idea and are feeling a bit unsure, talk about it to people you trust. Putting it out into the world is the first step, and having people you trust around you to pick you up and support you can help you start believing in yourself.
- Sometimes it's about having an idea, writing it down, sleeping on it, coming back to it and seeing if it goes anywhere. Sometimes it will. Sometimes it won't. But keep hold of it whilst you work that out.
- I know it's hard, but try not to rely on someone else to make you feel better about yourself. We all love compliments (we're only human), but starting to believe in yourself can lift you when someone else isn't there to do it.
- Practise conviction! Start small ('I am working on this . . .', 'I would like to go here on Saturday . . .'). Having conviction when talking about something means you'll almost certainly be met with someone responding in a positive way.
- When you feel like a fraud or an imposter, try and keep it schtum from the big cheeses – you're so much better than your imposter syndrome, so don't do yourself a disservice.
- Remember: the best way to eat an elephant is one small bite at a time.

- If you never try it or put it out there, you can never improve on it. You can never get better at something if you never start it.
- Don't hold on to guilt about every mistake you've ever made.
- Don't downplay your successes. You've worked hard to achieve them; don't make them seem smaller than they are for fear of not coming across how you want.
- Treat situations as if they belonged to a friend. If you'd say it to a friend, then say it to yourself too.
- Practise some TLC. Do more of what you want to feel confident in – if that means more books, more dancing and more weekend baking, then so be it!

Life After the Club

You're always welcome back

In an ideal world, perhaps there wouldn't be the need for a club celebrating (or reclaiming) the big old word that is insecurity. But I've discovered it's something that affects us all. Whether it's from a fleeting moment in the mirror whilst getting ready for work, or a quick scroll on our social media platform of choice, it can feel all-encompassing.

I'm certainly no expert, but one thing I do know is that insecurities don't go away. They develop, shift and change with age, and by building a tackle-it toolkit from today we can learn to manage it from the outset. Some of us are proud to speak up about our insecurities and can embrace them like an old friend – but often, we try to cover them up like a mountainous new spot before a presentation, or hide them away because we're too embarrassed to admit we have them.

It's not easy, and it doesn't come overnight, but with a bit of practice we can master the day-to-day insecurities and get by with a more self-cheerleading and self-compassionate outlook, which means we won't need to wait for others to give us the big high-five because we can do it for ourselves.

With any luck, this club isn't something you'll need to be a part of forever, but hopefully the assurance that it's always here, for the bad days and the good, will be enough to pick you up when you need it most.

If you're ever in doubt, here are the key takeaways from the book – in case you don't have time to riffle through the pages as you rush out of the front door, but just need a quick shot of feel-good, or a small reminder for the day going forward. Remember, we're here for you – and there's probably another one of us experiencing the same thing at this very moment . . .

If in doubt, don't forget:
- You're never alone in this. Whether you're feeling totally flat, comparing yourself or giving yourself grief for not achieving something you thought you should've, everyone has had to deal with this too at some point – even the people you admire the most.
- If you can't bring yourself to unfollow, mute anybody on social media that doesn't make you feel happy, inspired or full of beans. Life is far too short to spend time indulging in social media pages that don't make you feel good.
- Take care of yourself the way you would your

best friend, or a four-year-old version of you. Listen to your body and look after it as if it were a mission on your favourite PlayStation game.

- Pay attention to the way you talk to and about your body. Check your language and make sure it's kind at best and neutral at average.
- Look after your friendships like you would the flowers in your garden (after splashing out at the garden centre).
- The most important opinion is the one you have of yourself. You will never be able to change what other people think of you – so instead work on how you think of yourself.
- If you never try it, you can never get better at it.
- Finally, know that you can't pour from an empty cup. It's OK to take a break sometimes and speak to someone about it. You're not supposed to be able to do it all at 100 mph all of the time. You are one person. Look after yourself, always.

' . . . and please love yourself! (Said my mum at the end of a call.)'

Maria, Oxford

The Insecure Girl's Library

If you want to add a bit of sunshine to your feed, laughter to your listening, or just a bit of go-get-'em pizzazz to your everyday, here are some additional resources that I turn to again and again ('further reading', if we want to be proper about it).

INSTAGRAM

For the ultimate pick-me-up, I recommend:

- @alifemoreinspired
- @amaliah_com
- @ashlukadraws
- @britandco
- @cawligraphy
- @charliebcuff
- @emilycoxhead
- @frances_quinn

- @girlsnightinclub
- @gurlstalk
- @heysuperstar
- @iamlaurajackson
- @jamie_windust
- @jessiecave
- @khadijah_mellah
- @listen.louder
- @lucysheridan
- @lvernon2000
- @martinamartian
- @mikaelaloach
- @naomishimada
- @r29unbothered
- @stacieswift
- @thisisaliceskinner
- @thissarahpowell
- @tylerfeder

Body anxiety getting you down? These ladies champion all things wonderful about us:

- @abis_acne
- @antidietriotclub
- @bethany_rutter
- @beyondbeautifulbook
- @bodyposipanda
- @bryonygordon
- @calliethorpe

- @carlyfindlay
- @celestebarber
- @theconfidencecorner
- @enamasiama
- @girlswillbeboys_
- @gynaegeek
- @iamdaniadriana
- @itstrinanicole
- @i_weigh
- @jess_megan_
- @nadia.craddock
- @nerdabouttown
- @pink_bits
- @rollinfunky
- @rubyrare
- @scarrednotscared
- @skinnoshame
- @stylemesunday
- @talontedlex
- @the.vulva.gallery
- @torie_snelvis

Awe-inspiring activists to help you feel informed (or if you want to make a change):

- @100womeniknow
- @africabrooke
- @bbcbodypositive
- @charlie_craggs

- @deebaalinasyed
- @disgracecampbell
- @emsladedmondson
- @florencegiven
- @ginamartin
- @goddessplatform
- @gretathunberg
- @hellomynameiswednesday
- @howtoglitteraturd
- @iamlaurenmahon
- @knickers_models_own
- @laurathomasphd
- @monachalabi
- @nafisa_bakkar
- @nataliebyrne
- @novareidofficial
- @reshmasaujani
- @saimathompson
- @scarcurtis
- @tollydollyposh

FOR YOUR BOOKSHELF

Be The Change – Gina Martin
Beyond Beautiful – Anuschka Rees
Big Magic – Elizabeth Gilbert
Comfort Zones – edited by Sonder & Tell

Eat Up! – Ruby Tandoh
How to Be a Grown-Up – Daisy Buchanan
I Will Not Be Erased – gal-dem
Just Eat It – Laura Thomas
Life Honestly – The Pool
More Than Enough – Elaine Welteroth
Playing Big – Tara Mohr
Reasons to Stay Alive – Matt Haig
Sorry I'm Late, I Didn't Want to Come – Jessica Pan
The Comparison Cure – Lucy Sheridan
The Discomfort Zone – Farrah Storr

TOP OF THE PODS

Bryony Gordon's Mad World
Ctrl Alt Delete – Emma Gannon
Desert Island Discs
Happy Place – Fearne Cotton
Honestly Podcast with Clemmie Telford
How To Fail with Elizabeth Day
Nobody Panic – Tessa Coates and Stevie Martin
The Fringe of It (absolutely not biased!) – Charlotte
    Jacklin and Liv Purvis
The Guilty Feminist – Deborah Frances-White
The Gurls Talk Podcast – Adwoa Aboah
The Receipts Podcast – Tolani 'Tolly T' Shoneye, Milena
    Sanchez and Audrey Akande

Things You Can't Ask Yer Mum – Lizzy Hadfield and
  Lindsey Holland
Wobble – Jules von Hep and Sarah Powell

AND THE APPS

Bumble BFF – Connect, network and make new friends.

Calm – Meditation and sleep-aid app, with everything from breathing and meditation exercises to bedtime stories.

Flora: Focus & Study in Forest – A goal- and habit-tracking app that helps you keep your phone use down. Plant a seed on the app, and as you focus on your goals it grows into a tree.

Happy Not Perfect – A 'happiness workout' app that offers meditations, coaching sessions and ways of releasing your worries.

Moment – A screen time control app, to track usage on your phone.

Peanut – Meet and connect with like-minded mums locally.

Acknowledgements

I didn't think anything could instill clammy hands and moderate panic in me like driving, talking in front of a group of more than four or having to cancel plans after email tennis. Alas, writing an acknowledgements page for the book I never thought I'd be fortunate enough to write, and forgetting anyone, must top it.

I'm probably the millionth person to make an Oscars speech joke on this page (so, I, ugh, won't) but apologies in advance for this. I got very overexcited but really, you're just lucky I didn't include the DPD deliveryman too.

Anyway, to Mum, Dad and baby George. The most supportive, loving, thoughtful and wonderful people you could ever wish to meet. Thank you for nipping insecurity in the bud at every opportunity for me, teaching me what it is to be kind and selfless, for making me laugh endlessly and being my best friends, as well as family. Also, to Nanny Janet, Granddad Graham, Granddad Fred and Nanny Joan for the phone calls, life-lessons and being the biggest fanclub I could wish for (and teaching me what it is to grow old(er) gracefully). You are the best family a girl could wish for.

To Joe. For listening to my worries, keeping me updated with the best dog tweets, making me tea on tap and drying my tears when I've ever felt like I couldn't do this. You've helped with everything you could (percentages!) and been the biggest support and love I could ask for. And obviously Maggie (can I thank my dog? Is that . . . a bit odd?). (Thanks Maggie, regardless.)

To my best friend Gemma, and my incredible friends Genevieve, Daisy, Carrie, as well as my sisters, Molly and Lucy, for being patient, making my stomach ache from laughter and always being the rocks I needed. Thanks for not losing all hope in me when I took weeks to text back (this is why)! (But you knew that!) Plus all of my other incredible pals (you know who you are) who have supplied all the cuddles, warmth and support that I couldn't have done without. I don't know what I did to deserve you all.

To the bestest literary agents, Abigail and Megan, for having faith in me from day dot, and never making me feel intimidated by your collective coolness. You made me feel capable and like an ACTUAL IRL WRITER when I did not. So thank you. Thank you to my incredible agent Tilly (and family at Storm too) who always believed in me (even when I didn't). I am incredibly fortunate to have you.

The b i g g e s t thank you to my editor Ru (and Emily) and everyone at my amazing publisher Orion who not only believed this book would be a good idea, but have been the most brilliant team of women to work with (I hope you won't mind me still coming in for pastry meetings on the roof when this is finally out). You instilled so much faith in me, and I can't thank you enough for trusting me with this.

Acknowledgements

Thank you to the wonderful contributors who gave their time, knowledge and wisdom to these pages – Africa, Lucy, Nadia, Megan, Sarah, Kate, Deeba and Saima – you are all beyond inspiring, and it is a privilege to have you in these pages. Thank you to all of the incredible people who answered survey questions and shared experiences for these pages too – you have made this book what it is and I wish I could have included every story. I am so grateful.

Nearly there . . . To Charlotte, for being the greatest editorial assistant and making sure the club was ticking over with amazing content and stories when I was writing this book. I've never met someone so organised, thoughtful and committed to the wonders of pop music. You are a star.

And finally, you: the women vulnerable, brave and generous enough to share your stories over on The Insecure Girls' Club in the first place. When I started this club I had no idea of what it could be, and without you all, it wouldn't be much at all. I have been floored by the kindness, support, cupcakes(!) and words, and hope this book has done you all justice. Thank you. (I did it!)

Notes

1 'Esquire Meets Emma Watson', *Esquire* (April 2016)
2 'Beyoncé in Her Own Words', *Vogue* (September 2018)
3 *Becoming*, Michelle Obama (Viking, 2018)
4 'Actress Meryl Streep on films, fear and that Trump comment', *Yours* (June 2017)
5 'Real Girls, Real Pressure: A National Report on the State of Self-Esteem', The Dove Self-Esteem Fund (June 2008)
6 'Alexa Chung on love, life lessons and building her fashion empire', *ES Magazine* (December 2016)
7 'Ads Everywhere: The Race to Grab Your Brain', *Psychology Today* (November 2012)
8 The Girlguiding Girls' Attitudes Survey 2018
9 Ibid.
10 *Playing Big*, Tara Mohr (Gotham Books, 2014)
11 'Unhooking from Praise and Criticism with Tara Mohr', *Design Sponge* (March 2016)
12 'The Woman Who Wasn't There: Converging evidence that subliminal social comparison affects self-evaluation', *Journal of Experimental Social Psychology* (November 2017)

13 *Beta: Quiet Girls Can Run the World*, Rebecca Holman (Coronet, 2017)

14 OnePoll survey for *Access Commercial Finance* (June 2018)

15 Russell Brand on Instagram: https://www.instagram.com/p/Bu4djEkHDJO/

16 *How to Be a Grown-Up*, Daisy Buchanan (Headline, 2017)

17 'Body image: How we think and feel about our bodies', Mental Health Foundation with YouGov (March 2019)

18 'The Curate Escape', YMCA (May 2019)

19 'Working in fashion gave me such crippling body anxiety, I quit', *Metro* (May 2019)

20 Davina McCall on Fearne Cotton's *Happy Place* https://player.fm/series/happy-place/davina-mccall

21 *Beyond Beautiful*, Anuschka Rees (Ten Speed Press, 2019)

22 'Beyoncé in Her Own Words', ibid.

23 'Taking Part focus on: social media', Department for Culture, Media and Sport statistical release (April 2016)

24 'Women's Bragging Rights: Overcoming Modesty Norms to Facilitate Women's Self-Promotion', *Psychology of Women Quarterly* (2013)

25 'Why You Should Talk To Strangers', Kio Stark TED talk (2016)

26 'Half of your friends lost in seven years', *Netherlands Organization for Scientific Research* (May 2009)

27 'Lifetime of loneliness', Young Women's Trust survey (June–July 2018)

28 RBS survey with YouGov (February 2019) https://www.rbs.com/rbs/news/2019/04/one-in-five-adults-in-scotland-

identify-monday-as-the-most-stres.html

29 *The Five Love Languages*, Gary Chapman (Northfield Publishing, 1992)

30 'Thirty Things I've Learned at Thirty', Lucy Williams for *Fashion Me Now* (February 2017)

31 *How to Be a Grown-Up*, ibid.

32 *Life Honestly*, The Pool (Bluebird, 2018)

About the Author

Olivia has been a freelance fashion and lifestyle writer and blogger for nigh on a decade. After starting her blog, *What Olivia Did*, in 2010, she went on to win the Cosmopolitan Blog Award for best newcomer. In 2014 she went full-time with the blog, introducing YouTube to her repertoire with videos ranging from style, beauty and interviews to travel. This earned her a nomination for Best YouTuber at the Glamour Women of the Year Awards in 2017. She also co-hosts the popular podcast *The Fringe of It* with Charlotte Jacklin and started The Insecure Girls' Club in late 2018.